Praise for *Recovery from Trauma, Addiction, or Both*

"This is a terrific book. Lucid and eminently practical, it summarizes what Dr. Najavits has learned helps patients in over three decades of practice and research. Page upon page, she helps you confront what is going on inside of yourself. It's a step-by-step road to recovery from the enslavement of trauma and addiction. This is the sort of book you put by your bedside to visit over and over again as a guide to dealing with numbing, addiction, the secrets you try to keep from yourself, and underlying issues. I cannot recommend this book highly enough."

—*Bessel A. van der Kolk, MD, author of* The Body Keeps the Score

"In 13 years of recovery in AA, I often heard the refrain 'I never got the instruction manual on life.' Well, this book by Lisa Najavits might just be the only instruction book on recovery you'll ever need! It shines with a fresh perspective, jargon-free writing, and vivid personal inspiration in an overpopulated field."

—*Frank F., New York City*

"In this remarkable book, Dr. Najavits speaks to diverse audiences in a way that is clear, practical, and deeply engaging. She offers an unflinching look at the challenges of working on trauma and addiction, while always conveying a message of hope. People struggling with either or both issues will find a path to improve their life. Professionals too can use this as a companion to therapy, allowing patients to extend their efforts through a flexible but carefully structured process."

—*Joan E. Zweben, PhD, Executive Director, East Bay Community Recovery Project, Oakland, California; staff psychologist, San Francisco VA Medical Center*

"A welcome contribution. Dr. Najavits provides a comprehensive framework for recovery. She has woven her extensive clinical experience with the voices of people in recovery to create a rich and accessible resource."

—*Stephanie S. Covington, PhD, LCSW, author of* A Woman's Way through the Twelve Steps

"Many times in AA (or 'the rooms'), I have heard someone say, 'It's the language of the heart; what comes from the heart reaches the heart.' This work exemplifies that thought while also staying true to itself with structure and advice for addicts and trauma survivors. But more than going through the steps of recovery, Dr. Najavits shows how to do so with dignity and pride in what you may accomplish. I never felt alone while reading this book."

—*David T., Washington, DC*

RECOVERY FROM TRAUMA, ADDICTION, OR BOTH

Also by Lisa M. Najavits

A Woman's Addiction Workbook
(New Harbinger Publications)

For professionals

Seeking Safety: A Treatment Manual for PTSD and Substance Abuse
(The Guilford Press)

Recovery from Trauma, Addiction, or Both

Strategies for Finding Your Best Self

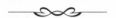

LISA M. NAJAVITS, PhD

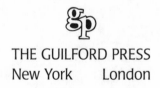

THE GUILFORD PRESS
New York   London

Published by The Guilford Press
A Division of Guilford Publications, Inc.
370 Seventh Avenue, Suite 1200, New York, NY 10001
www.guilford.com

The information in this volume is not intended as a substitute for consultation with health care professionals. Each individual's health concerns should be evaluated by a qualified professional.

Printed in the United States of America

This book is printed on acid-free paper.

Last digit is print number: 9   8   7   6   5   4   3   2   1

Library of Congress Cataloging-in-Publication Data is available from the publisher.

ISBN: 978-1-4625-2198-2 (paper) – ISBN: 978-1-4625-3030-4 (cloth)

The quotations in this book from people in recovery are used with permission and/or were created from composites, with identifying details disguised to protect privacy.

Contents

List of Exercises ix

Preface xi

1   Moving forward from trauma, addiction, or both 1

2   Starting out 9

3   "Things turn out okay" – David's experience 19

4   It's medical – you're not crazy, lazy, or bad 23

5   How do people change? 35

6   The world is your school 45

7   Listen to your behavior 47

8   Wish versus reality 55

9   Find your way 61

10 Possible selves 72

11 The language of trauma and addiction 78

12 Safe coping skills 86

13 Social pain 91

14 True self-compassion 97

15 Why trauma and addiction go together 103

16 Forgiving yourself 112

17 Body and biology 117

18   Getting to a calm place: The skill of *grounding*   125

19   The culture of silence   131

20   Motivation: Leverage one problem to help another   136

21   Tip the Scales recovery plan   141

22   Every child is a detective   150

23   How to survive a relapse   155

24   See the link   158

25   Practice   162

26   Identity: How you view yourself   166

27   Perception: How others view you   172

28   The decision to grow   179

29   Dark feelings: Rage, hatred, revenge, bitterness   186

30   Imagination   195

31   Create a healing image   201

32   Find a good counselor   206

33   Two types of trauma counseling   214

34   What the wounded can give back   222

35   "We are all in the gutter, but some of us are looking at the stars" 226

Appendix A. How others can help – family, friends, partners,   231
sponsors, counselors

Appendix B. Resources   250

Appendix C. Excessive Behavior Scale   256

Appendix D. Brief quiz on trauma and addiction: Knowledge is power   261

References   269

Index   273

About the Author   277

List of Exercises

Do you have trauma problems?   28

Do you have an addiction problem?   32

Is it safe or unsafe?   48

The Safe Behavior Scale   51

The good that comes from facing your truth   58

12 questions to ask when seeking help   69

Your possible selves   74

Addiction language   79

Trauma language   81

The Scavenger Hunt Game   83

The Safe Coping Skills List   86

How do you score on compassion?   100

Your patterns of trauma, addiction, or both   109

Self-forgiveness   114

Your relationship with your body   121

Try out grounding   126

Your motivation   138

Create your Tip the Scales recovery plan   142

Choose the messages you want to keep   151

The link between addiction and trauma in the present   158

How would you cope . . . ?   162

Encourage yourself to grow   181

Play with your recovery imagination   195

Create your healing image   203

Evaluate your counseling   208

Quiz: Two types of trauma counseling   219

And you?   227

Preface

The purpose of this book is to help you find your best self, which may be buried, sometimes quite deeply, amid layers of trauma, addiction, or both.

For over 25 years I've listened to, encouraged, and witnessed the recovery work of people who have struggled with these issues. Each chapter is a small expression of what I've learned from them as well as what's known in the professional field.

Because I can't sit with you and hear your story, I've included two features to help bring this book closer to such a direct connection.

First, I've tried to make it as interactive as possible with reflection points and exercises to ask you the kinds of questions we would explore if we were working together in counseling. Just as in actual counseling, you can choose to answer these or not. The goal is to help you understand yourself better and feel more compassion for yourself so that you can take action. When I picture you reading this book, I envision that here or there you'll be sparked by something that moves you, which may help you grow or at least get through the next tough moment. For that to occur, what you read needs to engage both your head and your heart (and your spirit, if you believe in that) so that this book is not a dry, abstract experience.

Second, and what may be the most important aspect of this book for some, are the quotes from people in recovery from trauma and addiction. This book took me several years to write in part because after I "finished" it, something was clearly missing. (I owe thanks here to David, whom you'll meet in Chapter 3, and Kitty Moore at The Guilford Press, both of whom pointed this out.) I decided to bring it to life by asking people in recovery to read a chapter and write or talk to me about how it relates to their recovery. Each of these people – who are wide-ranging in their life history as well as age, gender, ethnicity, and geography – did it to be of service to others.

So think of this book as a community of support. Each of us is rooting for you and hoping you'll do all you can to get better. And if there's one thing you'll hear across their words and mine it's that you *can* get better, even if that goal seems unreachable, as remote as a far-off planet.

To make your process as easy as possible, each chapter is brief and offers one way forward relevant to trauma, addiction, or both. You can read the chapters in any order and as few or as many as you choose; each is independent of the others. You can decide what to work on, at your own pace, combined with any other available supports and treatments. Recovery is creative; it's about trying options and figuring out what fits for you. It's about taking what's good about you, your talents and capacities, and directing them toward improving parts of your life that aren't working. It's about experiments, each moving you a bit closer to your goals. There's no one way; hold on to what works and let go of the rest. Strive to launch what's deepest and best within you.

This book also reflects changes in health care for trauma and addiction. These issues have typically been addressed separately. It's been a major shift, a sort of mini-revolution, to address both at the same time when people have both. Numerous counselors, programs, peers, researchers, and policymakers have enacted this shift by listening closely to the needs of people with addiction and trauma. This book is rooted in that important work. The chapters derive from evidence-based practice, which means they draw from a mix of research and clinical innovation. I've been privileged to have had a career in that field at Harvard Medical School and McLean Hospital for 25 years; at Boston University School of Medicine and the Veterans Affairs Boston Healthcare System for 12 years; and with numerous collaborations with colleagues at other universities and programs. A counseling approach I developed, Seeking Safety, became a widely used, evidence-based model for co-occurring trauma and addiction, and I've been privileged to be part of a team that has trained tens of thousands of counselors in it around the country and the world. I've been moved by the exceptional dedication of those who are trying to improve the lives of those with addiction and trauma problems from so many different types of painful experiences: domestic violence, war, homelessness, child abuse, terrorism, natural disasters, crime, and others.

I have long wanted to write a self-help book because I've seen how people can get better if they're given enough of even small doses of inspiration, practical advice, new ideas, and education. I've included these in equal measure in the hope that there's something here for everyone. Yet sending a book into the world is not a light matter when taking on the tall task of trying to help people help themselves. I'm acutely aware that a book such as this is small ballast relative to the enormity of trauma and addiction.

The larger context is a humbling one. Rates of trauma and addiction remain far too high and appear to be increasing throughout the world. Most people with trauma and addiction never get professional help. Recovery needs to be continually fought for, both individually and collectively, as part of a public health mission that continues to grow over time. The field is still young, and much more needs to be learned and shared.

Before closing here, I have many people to thank. I am deeply grateful to those who offered their recovery stories for this book – David C., Bev P., Katrina Z., Jennifer, Shoshi, Jennyfer Gordon, and to those who chose to stay anonymous. My sincere thanks also go to some of the many colleagues who keep me inspired: Summer Krause, Brenda Underhill, Gabriella Grant, Kay Johnson, Martha Schmitz, Joni Utley, Sarah Gentry, Cary Smith, Denise Hien, Teresa Marsh, Sermed Alkass, Lily Awad, David Deitch, Hein de Haan, Tony Dekker, Joan Zweben, and Marge Cramer. Extra special recognition is due to the first four and to Jennifer Perlman, David C., Shoshi, Katrina Z., and Mary B., for providing detailed feedback on the manuscript.

My forever-love goes to Burke Nersesian, Paul Lewis, and Judy Najavits for their day-to-day presence in such joyful and amazing ways.

And thank you, Fran Williams, for sending me this quote:

"Life will break you. Nobody can protect you from that, and living alone won't either, for solitude will also break you with its yearning. You have to love. You have to feel. It is the reason you are here on earth. You are here to risk your heart. You are here to be swallowed up. And when it happens that you are broken, or betrayed, or left, or hurt, or death brushes near, let yourself sit by an apple tree and listen to the apples falling all around you in heaps, wasting their sweetness. Tell yourself you tasted as many as you could."
 —From *The Painted Drum* by Louise Erdrich, Native American writer
 and winner of the National Book Award

RECOVERY FROM TRAUMA, ADDICTION, OR BOTH

1

Moving forward
from trauma, addiction, or both

I am not what happened to me. I am what I choose to become.
—CARL GUSTAV JUNG, 20th-century Swiss psychiatrist and writer

You can heal from trauma and addiction. In the words of people who have done it:

Living with addiction [or trauma] "is sort of like growing up on a boat. The ground is always moving underneath you, sometimes you learn to stay upright, when the water is gentle, but at times it's completely impossible, and it's all you can do to lie flat and hang on for dear life. Coming into recovery . . . it's like washing up on the shore and standing up. Even though you're on solid ground, it takes a while to stop reeling and constantly counterbalancing, because that's all you know. People on land might look at you like you're insane for hanging on to a railing, because they've always stood on solid ground and can't understand being that involuntarily imbalanced. Over time, you start to gain your land legs, though, and stop having to reel back and forth just to stay upright. Then you wake up one day and realize that you can walk a straight line on dry land for the first time. You always remember the buck and roll and learning to walk again, but you learn to stay upright and walk among the 'land people.' "
—From *www.soberrecovery.com*

"Living in recovery is like gradually waking up from a long, nightmare-filled sleep. It is discovering pale days slowly fading into warm, colorful transforming experiences rich with meaning and joy."

Emotional pain that you've carried, even for a long time, can become the seed of growth.

Trauma and Addiction

Throughout the world, trauma and addiction are two of the most difficult and common issues that people face.

Trauma Means "Wound"

Trauma comes from the Greek word for *wound,* which vividly describes what it feels like. It's a serious, unwanted, harmful event that can lead to lasting pain. The wounds may be physical, emotional, or both. Most people endure at least one in their lifetime and some have a lot of them.

The definition of *trauma* from the American Psychiatric Association (2013) refers to physical events such as the following:

■ car accident ■ sexual assault ■ military combat ■ physical violence ■ fire ■ hurricane, tornado, or other natural disaster ■ terrorist incident ■ life-threatening illness or injury ■ sudden death of someone close to you ■ industrial accident ■ domestic violence

---

"Starting at the moment that the bomb went off, I had a mental video and audio of that day's experiences that played 24 hours a day, along with everything else I was doing."
—Paul Heath, survivor of the Oklahoma City bombing, in *Learning to Live Past 9:02 am, April 19, 1995,* by Kathryn Foxhall

---

Trauma can also refer to deeply disturbing experiences that are not physical in nature:

■ emotional abuse ■ bullying ■ growing up with mentally ill parents ■ neglect ■ abandonment ■ homelessness ■ major loss ■ severe social rejection ■ ongoing serious stress, such as chronic pain, poverty, or discrimination

✧ Have you had trauma?

How trauma occurs also matters. It can happen ...

> » *To a person or entire communities.* Whole cultures can suffer trauma as in genocide and slavery, which carries forward emotionally over generations.
> » *Amid support or brutality.* Humiliation, silence, betrayal, and blame worsen the impact of trauma.
> » *Directly or threatened or witnessed.* For example, a child may see violence happening to a parent.
> » *Once or often.* Some people say there were "too many times to remember."

Whatever your history of trauma, you can learn new ways to cope with it. The past can't be rewritten, but you can change how you relate to it.

Addiction Means "Can't Stop"

Addiction comes from Latin roots for *enslavement,* which perfectly describes what serious addiction feels like. But addiction can be mild, moderate, or severe. You don't have to fit the image of an addict to have a problem. It can creep up on you without your noticing. Others may see it before you do. Or you may have a problem that's not yet a full-blown addiction.

Broadly, addiction means that *you keep engaging in a behavior despite the harm it causes.* You keep drinking even though your doctor tells you to stop. You keep gambling despite your debt. You keep having affairs even if it costs you relationships. People without addiction would stop to preserve their health, finances, or relationships. People with addiction keep repeating the behavior. They may want to stop but can't. They feel more and more out of control. Or they may think it's not a problem, but the facts show that it is.

"In those rare times lately when I sit back and take stock of myself, I can see that I'm spending hour after hour, evenings and weekends, just sitting around staring at porn. Instead of actually having 'a life,' I've lost precious hours, days, weeks, months, even years in isolation and loneliness. Most days I can't wait for work to end so I can get home to my porn collection. Whoever says this problem doesn't exist should try walking in my shoes for a few days.... I don't know what it is to have a real relationship because all I've ever experienced is webcam hookups and porn."
—From *Always Turned On: Sex Addiction in the Digital Age,* by Robert Weiss and Jennifer P. Schneider

---

Substance addiction – alcohol or drugs – is one of the most common addictions and also the most studied. The formal term is *substance use disorder,* and 15% of people develop it in their lifetime. In the United States it's the second most common psychological problem after depression. Drug overdoses currently kill more Americans than cars or guns.

But people can get addicted to all sorts of behaviors, including gambling, pornography, sex, work, food, spending or shopping, electronics (such as television, Internet, texting, and gaming), rage, violence, self-harm such as cutting or burning, and body-related behavior such as plastic surgery, tattooing, tanning, or exercise. These *behavioral addictions* are becoming more and more recognized as they seem to have many of the same features as substance addiction.

✧ Are there any behaviors you want to reduce – alcohol, drugs, gambling, eating, spending, or any others?

A New Perspective Linking Trauma and Addiction

A major breakthrough in recent years is the understanding of how common it is for *both* trauma and addiction to happen to the same person.

Sometimes trauma leads to addiction, sometimes addiction leads to trauma, and sometimes both occur at the same time. For most people trauma occurs first, then addiction – often through an attempt to try to cope with emotional or physical pain. This pattern has existed throughout history, including the description here by a famous 19th-century writer.

"I have absolutely no pleasure in the stimulants in which I sometimes so madly indulge. It has not been in the pursuit of pleasure that I have periled life and reputation and reason. It has been in the desperate attempt to escape from torturing memories . . . from a sense of insupportable loneliness and a dread of some strange impending doom."
—From the letters of Edgar Allan Poe

It makes perfect sense that people reach for something to try to feel better when they're distressed. A trauma survivor may drink to deal with nightmares or binge to soothe inner pain. People abuse substances, gamble away their money, overeat, work too hard, and spend too much because they want to shift feelings. They may want to feel *more* of something, such as energy, joy, or calm; or *less* of something, such as rage, hurt, loneliness, or self-hatred. Feelings get thrown off balance due to trauma. You may have no feeling (numb) or too much feeling (overwhelmed) or bounce back and forth between these. Addictive behavior can "solve" trauma problems in the short term even though it's destructive in the long term.

To those who don't understand, addiction is often judged as bad rather than seen at a deeper level as an attempt to cope. The truth is that even though addictive behavior causes problems, it may have been safer in the moment than the alternative. Some people say substance use calmed them enough to prevent suicide or helped them survive abuse they couldn't escape.

Jennyfer: "I probably would have committed suicide if I hadn't turned to drugs as a way to cope after my accident – that fateful moment when a stray bullet in the night altered the course of my life forever. I think a lot about my life since my traumatic brain injury – my choices, addictions, the insane risks I have taken, and my absolute lack of fear. I have hopped on planes and relocated to foreign countries where I didn't know a soul, because I felt like there was an invisible driving force whispering in my ear, 'All you have is today.'"

The goal now is to find ways to cope with trauma so that you won't need addictive behavior. But you can honor that you may have used it to survive emotionally or physically.

Before Getting into Recovery versus After

Notice what people say before they get into recovery versus after.

Before recovery

- "I'm haunted by my memories." - "I drink to get to sleep at night." - "I have urges to hurt myself." - "I'm numb." - "I don't take care of my body." - "I hate myself." - "When I use, it decreases the rage." - "I'm with a partner who hits me." - "When I have flashbacks, I go to the casino to calm down." - "Cocaine gives me permission to feel sexual." - "I drink to keep from killing myself." - "Heroin is the only way I know to nurture myself." - "When I drink, I cry about all the things that happened to me." - "I can't stop doing what I do." - "I feel scared a lot." - "Using drugs closes the door to my past." - "I feel like a failure." - "A food binge makes me feel better."

✧ Do any of those statements sound familiar to you?

In recovery

▪ "I'm no longer afraid of my memories." ▪ "When I get cravings to use, I can let them pass." ▪ "I am better at choosing people who treat me well." ▪ "I no longer feel angry all the time." ▪ "Things that used to throw me – I'd be in bed for days, depressed – I can handle now." ▪ "I can be sexual without getting triggered." ▪ "I learned that I don't have to rebel to be seen and heard." ▪ "Now I view my addiction as a medical illness." ▪ "For the first time, I can forgive myself. I really feel it – it's not just words." ▪ "I know who I am; I'm not a stranger to myself anymore." ▪ "I take care of my body now." ▪ "I became a good mother to my kids the more I became nurturing toward myself." ▪ "I stopped keeping secrets." ▪ "I understand now that I don't have to suffer so much." ▪ "After being down for so long, hating myself, I don't take for granted what it feels like to be up. There's a sense of appreciation." ▪ "I can say what I want rather than blowing up." ▪ "Now other people are more important to me than drugs."

✧ Which statements sound like what you want for yourself?

The Old Way – Split Worlds: Trauma *or* Addiction

Imagine that you're seeking help for addiction plus a history of painful trauma – perhaps childhood physical, sexual, and emotional abuse; a serious car accident; or combat. In traditional addiction approaches, you might be told to "Get clean and sober first" or "Just work on your addiction recovery." You may think, "No one wants to hear what happened," "I'm weak for focusing on it," or "Maybe what I went through wasn't that important." There may be caring people who want to help, but perhaps they were trained to avoid focusing on trauma.

So too if you have trauma problems, you might enter a mental health program where they never ask about addiction unless it's severe, in which case they refer you to an addiction program. They may say, "Come back when you've gotten the addiction under control" – a message that can leave you stuck, unable to address the trauma or the addiction successfully. One young woman, Chandra, said, "I had to hide my addiction to get into a trauma program. I lied because I knew that if I didn't get help for my PTSD I would never recover from substance abuse."

The worlds of trauma recovery and addiction recovery have historically been separate and largely remain so today. The two worlds have separate workforces, cultures, and funding. People with both trauma and addiction problems can get lost in the gap, rejected from help in one domain because they're too severe in the other.

Now imagine a new approach: you enter a program that's both *trauma-informed* and *addiction-informed*. You're asked about your trauma and addiction from the start, and the staff are trained to understand how each impacts the other. You're able to be open about both and learn skills to work on both at the same time, not delaying one for the other. You might feel more understood and more motivated to work on recovery. "It feels like it's a piece of the puzzle. There was a piece that was missing, and now it's not missing anymore," said one client in such a program.

Notice the differences between the old and new ways:

Focus on trauma *or* addiction	Focus on addiction *and* trauma
Traditional approach	New approach
Addiction is the focus or trauma is the focus, not both.	If you have both, you can get help for both.
"One size fits all" – there's one right way to heal.	"Many roads, one journey" – there are many ways to heal.
Attend one type of treatment.	Embrace all the help you can.
Work on addiction now and trauma later.	Work on both at the same time.
With addiction recovery you'll feel better and better.	Trauma problems may flare up as you maintain addiction recovery; this needs attention too.
If you heal trauma, the addiction will go away on its own.	Healing trauma alone is not enough.
If you work on trauma and addiction at the same time, you'll get worse.	It's *how* you work on it that matters. Working on both shows positive results if it's done well.
Addiction is just due to genes (biology).	Addiction is typically due to genes and environment (including trauma).
Lack of focus on gender or culture.	Gender and culture play a role in trauma and addiction.
Addictive behavior is an attempt to *avoid* trauma memories.	There are many reasons why people have addictive behavior.

One of the big moments in recovery is when you can see how trauma and addiction are linked if you have both issues. You open your heart and find ways to move forward. You tell a new story of who you are.

An Upward Spiral

Just as trauma and addiction are linked, so is their recovery. You can apply recovery skills to both at once, which is more powerful than working on each alone.

You can create an *upward spiral:* Improving one helps the other. In fact, people who have both issues prefer working on them together when they're given that option, research shows.

◇ What does the opening quote in this chapter mean to you?

◇ What feels hopeful for you right now?

RECOVERY VOICES

Lily – " . . . a life worth living"

Lily survived child abuse and had drug addiction that lasted into her 30s. "For so long I never thought about what I went through. Everything was a blur. All I lived for was to forget. Now I have a guiding light. When I crave a substance, it's a sign that there's something happening in my life that I need to pay attention to, a reminder of my past, a sign to change the story and practice taking care of me. It took me a long time to get to that. I didn't see the connection between my trauma and addiction. It was really hard to see it when I was living it. I couldn't escape the trauma when it was happening, and I wasn't going to give up the substances because it felt like that's what was saving my life at the time. I eventually landed in addiction treatment, and that helped, but it was silent about trauma. I was told that I shouldn't talk about it till later, but for me 'later' never came. Eventually I found a counselor who helped me work on both. He was really caring and also gave me ideas of what to try, a lot like what's in this book. I made it my mission to learn all I could. It wasn't a straight path; I still kept secrets. I gave up alcohol but lied about using pills. Or I'd have trauma nightmares and go back to alcohol. But over time I got stronger and more honest. The opening quote in this chapter captures what recovery means to me – yes, there's pain in life, but I can make choices that bring me more of what I want: love, good people, sobriety, and the adventure of life on life's terms. I can't change the past, but I have a life worth living."

2

Starting out

You don't have to see the whole staircase, just take the first step.
—Martin Luther King, Jr., 20th-century civil rights leader
  and Nobel Peace Prize winner

Recovery may be challenging, but this book is easy. You can start anywhere. Glance at the table of contents to see what intrigues you, read the chapters in order, or close your eyes and open to any page randomly. You can skip around . . . go fast or slow . . . focus in or just skim . . . do the exercises or not . . . read on your own or with someone else. You're the inventor of your recovery.

You can also use this book no matter where you are along your path. You may be just beginning, not sure you even have addiction or trauma problems. Or you may have years of solid recovery and want some fresh ideas to continue your work. You may have just addiction or trauma problems but not both, or you may have both but never worked on them together. You may have low-level problems and want to prevent them from getting worse, or you may have moderate or severe problems.

Throughout, you can set your own goals. For example, some people with addiction problems know they need to give up their addictive behavior completely (an *abstinence* approach); others want to start reducing it (*harm reduction*); some seek to return to safe levels of use (*controlled use*); and still others aren't sure of their goals and want help figuring out what's best for them. You'll be given honest advice about what may be best for you, given your history. You can also learn how to find good-quality professional care and self-help groups, which can further guide you in deciding what's best for you. This book is deeply respectful of the many different types of help out there, including Alcoholics Anonymous and other 12-step groups, SMART Recovery, and all types of professional help. This book can be used while you participate in any program or support. The more the better.

Also important is what you won't find here. You won't be asked to explore graphic details of trauma or addiction, which can be too upsetting, especially if you're early in recovery. Instead you'll find support that works within the context of a self-help book. In general, the material was designed to minimize triggers (reminders of trauma or addiction that set off intense feelings).

This chapter offers suggestions to help you get the most from this book so you can keep moving closer and closer to the person you want to be.

Consider Where You're at Now

You truly can start anywhere in the book right now. But if you'd like some guidance, explore the questions below. Take a look at each, as several may apply to you.

Are you unsure whether you have trauma or addiction?
See chapters that can help you figure that out: "It's medical – you're not crazy, lazy, or bad" (Chapter 4); "The language of trauma and addiction" (Chapter 11).

Do you have trauma or addiction, but not both?
Apply the ideas in this book to whichever one you do have.

Do you doubt that things can get better?
Focus on chapters that aim to inspire recovery: "Possible selves" (Chapter 10); "The decision to grow" (Chapter 28); "How do people change?" (Chapter 5); "The world is your school" (Chapter 6); "Motivation: Leverage one problem to help another" (Chapter 20); "Imagination" (Chapter 30).

Are you ready to work on recovery?
Start with some very practical chapters: "Safe coping skills" (Chapter 12); "Getting to a calm place: The skill of grounding" (Chapter 18); "Tip the Scales recovery plan" (Chapter 21).

Are you early in recovery?
Prioritize chapters that reinforce staying in recovery: "Create a healing image" (Chapter 31); "How to survive a relapse" (Chapter 23).

Do you want to understand more about the link between trauma and addiction?
See "Why trauma and addiction go together" (Chapter 15) and "See the link" (Chapter 24).

Do you want to deepen your recovery?
Consider "The culture of silence" (Chapter 19); "Social pain" (Chapter 13); "Every child is a detective" (Chapter 22); "Identity: How you view yourself" (Chapter 26); "Wish versus reality" (Chapter 8); "Perception: How others view you" (Chapter 27); "Dark feelings: Rage, hatred, revenge, bitterness" (Chapter 29).

Are you interested in treatment or support groups?
See "Find a good counselor" (Chapter 32); "Find your way" (Chapter 9); "Two types of trauma counseling" (Chapter 33).

Do you have caring people in your life?
Give them "How others can help – family, friends, partners, sponsors, counselors" (Appendix A).

Remember, all chapters are relevant no matter what your answers are to the questions above, so try to get to all chapters at least briefly.

Use Language That "Speaks" to You

Language is powerful. Use whatever words fit for you. *Trauma problems* is used in this book, but you can substitute *posttraumatic stress disorder* (PTSD) if you have that condition or use a general term such as *emotional pain*. *Addiction* occurs throughout, but you may not have a full-blown addiction and may prefer *problem behavior, excessive behavior, unsafe behavior,* or *addictive behavior.* Also this book focuses on all types of addiction, not just substances, so *addiction* and *using* can relate to any addictive behavior (*using alcohol, using gambling, using food, using sex,* etc.). This book refers to *recovery,* but you may prefer *healing, growth, progress,* or *change.* The key is not to get caught up in language, as that can be a way to stall recovery ("My partner says I'm an addict, but I know I'm not"). Just focus on the behaviors and feelings you want to change.

✧ Is there any language for *trauma, addiction,* or *recovery* that you prefer?

Stay Safe

With trauma and addiction, you may have difficulty protecting yourself from unsafe people and situations. Keep the following in mind.

Don't confront an abuser or any violent or dangerous person alone. Confronting unsafe people can evoke major backlash, including physical harm and verbal abuse. If you want to confront someone, do it carefully. Seek counselors, lawyers, or others who can guide you on how best to handle it.

Limit your access to weapons and sharps (knives, razors) if you have a history of harming yourself or others. The easier it is to access these, the more likely you are to use them.

Know where your local emergency room is and how you would get there. You may not need it, but being prepared helps if you have an urgent situation.

Avoid dangerous areas as much as you can. Don't walk alone at night in unsafe neighborhoods, for example. If you must go, try to have someone with you.

Keep a list of hotlines and other help available. See "Resources" (Appendix B) for such options, including for suicide prevention.

Block access to your addictive behavior as much as possible. Remove alcohol from the house, block gambling websites, and put unhealthy foods out of reach. If you're not yet ready to give up the behavior, do whatever you're willing to do now to delay it by making it harder to access.

Always carry identity and insurance cards. Also keep enough cash or a credit card so that you can get a ride or other help if needed.

Create a list of people to call for support. Store their phone numbers in "favorites" on your phone and put a list in your wallet so you can access them easily.

◇ What can you do to stay safe?

Create a Crisis Plan

A crisis plan is like insurance: you may not need it, but you want it to be there if something goes wrong. If you feel in danger of hurting yourself or anyone else and can't control the impulse, you *must* get help. Write down now who you would contact (emergency room, crisis center, hotline, counselor, partner, close friend), contact information for those people such as cell phone numbers, and other details. If you have a counselor or sponsor, get assistance in creating your plan. Also identify in advance how you'll handle a strong addiction craving or other problems even if they're not necessarily an emergency. Share your crisis plan with people you trust.

✧ What's your crisis plan?

Aim High, but Not for Perfection

Do all you can to heal, ending each day with a sense that you made a real effort. The more you prioritize healing and hold yourself to high standards, the faster you'll progress. However, you may find it hard to get motivated or may be so tough on yourself that nothing feels good enough. You may become so paralyzed by painful feelings that you can't do much at all. You may start out strong and then falter. These ups and downs are common, especially if you have severe trauma or addiction problems. So pace yourself. Allow for imperfection and keep refining as you go.

Consider Involving Others

You may want to engage others to support your recovery. Or you may prefer to wait until you have more people you can trust.

If you want to involve others, consider a counselor, friend, family member, 12-step sponsor, mentor, spiritual advisor, or peer. You can set up regular meeting times to go through a chapter at a time from this book with that person. You can also give the person a copy of "How others can help – family, friends, partners, sponsors, counselors" (Appendix A). If you're far enough along in recovery, you can even set up peer support self-help meetings with others who are working on trauma and/or addiction.

If you're trying to build more supportive people into your life, see the chapters in this book that focus on that: "Find your way" (Chapter 9); "Find a good counselor" (Chapter 32); "Two types of trauma counseling" (Chapter 33).

✧ Are there people you want to involve as you go through this book? If so, how do you want to involve them?

Leverage Your Strengths

Just as important as what's wrong is what's *right*. The more you grow your strengths, the more they offset your weaknesses.

» *Survival skills*: street smarts; practical wisdom.

» *Curiosity*: openness to new ideas and experiences.

» *Faith*: deep beliefs that help when times get tough.

» *Past success*: a record of achievements, which bodes well for future success.

» *People skills*: friendliness, humor, and charm; these build support and get others to help you.

» *Independence*: being resourceful, figuring things out, identifying options.

» *Intelligence*: the ability to learn.

» *Caring*: the capacity to love and dedicate yourself to people and meaningful causes in the world.

» *Self-awareness*: in touch with your feelings; aware of inner experiences; reflective; conscious.

» *Responsible*: able to hold a job, handle daily tasks, and stay organized.

» *Motivation*: energy and persistence; the gift of will; readiness to move forward.

» *Other strengths?* _____

✧ Circle your strengths in the list above.

✧ How can your strengths help you heal?

Remember That Trauma Can Be an Explanation, but Not an Excuse, for Addictive Behavior

This book takes a compassionate approach to trauma and addiction. But although trauma can be an *explanation* for addiction, it's not an *excuse* for it. This means that trauma can help you understand how addiction develops, but it's not an excuse to keep using. As anyone with addiction knows, *anything* can become a reason for using – "I had a hard day," "I deserve a good time," "My partner nags me," "The Red Sox won the World Series," "I got a promotion at work," "My kids are too loud," "It's my birthday." Trauma problems lead people to addictive behavior – this is a real and important fact. But it's not a rationale for continuing it. Learn to respond to your trauma problems without addictive behavior.

Also understand that resolving trauma problems doesn't mean you can simply return to behavior that was addictive for you in the past. You'll likely need to continue to manage it carefully.

Pamela had severe trauma and addiction to alcohol: "Did I drink too much, and did my drinking bring on more trauma, which caused all of the extra drinking that turned it from drinking to addiction? It really doesn't matter now, nor did it matter the day I got sober. But I still wonder about it, which leads me to a thought that maybe if I drank because of the trauma and I recover from the trauma, maybe I could drink without a problem. Hence I'm still an addict searching for a drink."

Protect Yourself from Triggers

Triggers are reminders of trauma or addiction that set off intense feelings that may be negative, such as anger or sadness, or positive, such as excitement or celebration. An addiction trigger might be seeing others drink or passing a bar or casino. A trauma trigger might be a smell or sound that reminds you of trauma. This book was written to avoid triggering material. You won't find vivid descriptions of addiction, trauma images, or other disturbing material. However, triggering can happen any time, and what's triggering for one person may not be for another. Do all you can to protect yourself from triggers, but know that triggering is common as you work on recovery. You may react strongly when reminded of trauma or addiction. Or you may have the opposite – numbness, no feeling – which is the flip side of triggering, a sort of safety valve in which your feelings shut down on their own because they're too intense. If you feel triggered, do whatever helps you in the moment to stay safe from acting on it. Distance from what triggered you, if possible. "Getting to a calm place: The skill of grounding" (Chapter 18) also provides ways to cope with triggers.

Note: "'Things turn out okay' – David's experience" (Chapter 3), is an inspiring story of a man's recovery from trauma and addiction. Although it's detailed, people who provided feedback on this book said it wasn't triggering for them.

Relate This Book to Your Life

The more you apply this book to your life, the more helpful it'll be. As you go along, mark sections you find meaningful. Notice your feelings: What moves you? What creates hope? Also, notice opportunities to engage more fully:

> » When you see a diamond icon ◇, it's an opportunity for reflection. These create a sort of dialogue such as might occur if you were sitting with a counselor or helpful friend.

> » When you see a star icon ✶ and the term *Explore,* it's an engaging exercise such as a brief quiz or a tool to evaluate where you're at.

You'll also find many quotations – an inspiring quote that starts each chapter and the Recovery Voices at the end of each chapter, which are quotes from people in recovery who share their experiences in relation to the chapter topic.

This book combines different ways of learning: through *emotion* (such as the quotations), *the mind* (ideas, knowledge), and *experience* (the exercises and reflections). The goal is to help you connect with what you're reading. You may also want to keep a journal to record insights that arise.

Focus on Your Recovery Goals

You may have specific goals that you want to achieve, such as decreasing trauma flashback, limiting substance use or other addictive behavior, developing better relationships, finding housing or a job, taking better care of your body, feeling less depressed, controlling your impulses, coming to terms with the past, and so on. You can apply this book to any such goals. Or you may not yet be clear what you want: trauma and addiction can narrow your ability to imagine your future. As you read, your goals will become more clear.

◇ What are your recovery goals at this point?

Respond to Your Needs

Many people share the experience of trauma and addiction, but differ in other ways. How long recovery takes and what will help you can vary based on . . .

» Your age, gender, culture, and personality.

» How severe your problems are. You may have mild addiction problems and severe trauma problems or vice versa. Your problems may be recent or long term; they may be ongoing or occasional.

» Additional challenges: in addition to trauma and/or addiction, you may need help with parenting, legal problems, medical problems such as chronic pain or HIV, anger, depression, or a disability, for example.

Whatever your needs, attend to them. Find as much help as possible. And apply the ideas in this book to problems beyond trauma and addiction. The more you actively work on your problems, the better you'll do.

✧ What current needs do you want help with?

Create a Routine for Working on This Book

Chaos and confusion are part of addiction and trauma. Counter these by creating a recovery routine that's the opposite of those: active, planned, paced, making steady progress. Try the following.

Set a reading target. A page a day or a chapter each week? It can be anything, as long as it's specific.

Try to make it the same each time. As much as possible, read this book at the same time each day, in the same location, and with the same people if you're doing it with others. Consistency eases the path.

Create reminders. Put it in your calendar as an appointment. Use email or text reminders. Your recovery is as important as any other appointments you have.

Make it visible. Put this book where you'll see it each day: in the middle of the floor, on the kitchen table, or next to your keys.

Do it even if you don't feel like it. One of the big myths about recovery is that you have to feel motivated to change. You don't. Motivation often comes later. You just need to take steps in the right direction. Make recovery reading part of your life like brushing your teeth – do it whether you feel like it or not.

Remember that any plan is better than no plan. Start with *any* plan that you think might work and then adjust it as you go.

◇ Are you willing to create a plan for using this book? What will it be?

Evaluate Your Progress

There are free validated measures that you can find online to track your progress. There are also mobile apps relevant to trauma and addiction to help with that. See "Resources" (Appendix B).

◇ When you look at the table of contents of this book, what chapters interest you most?

◇ Is there anything you can do to help yourself today?

◇ What increases your motivation for recovery?

RECOVERY VOICES

Leigh – "Take your time and be patient."

Leigh survived childhood physical and emotional abuse and later developed alcohol addiction. "I began my journey alone, and over 30 years later, my life is better than I could have ever dreamed. I was a high school dropout, and now I have completed my doctorate and own my own business. I have 30 years' sobriety and amazing friends I've made along the way. This chapter is a good reminder that it's so important to do all you can to get better. Recovery is hard work. And recovering from trauma and substance abuse is extremely hard work. My advice to someone starting out is: take your recovery seriously but remember to breathe every day. Take your time and be patient. If you change a little bit each week for the rest of your life, in just one year's time you will have made 52 changes. Walk through recovery with someone else; it may be a 12-step sponsor, a friend, or members from your group, but walk through it bravely. The change will be amazing, and although every day won't be perfect, it's one more day in recovery. Peace to you, my friend, and you never know who you may meet on your quest."

3

"Things turn out okay" – David's experience

The personal story below is real. David offered it here to help others.

Things turn out okay.

I'm not going to say things have a happy ending, because I have no idea what is in store for me, but I used to hate myself, I used to feel hopeless, I used to feel helpless (and worthless, stupid, and was fully addicted to any substance or behavior that could make me feel good, even if only for a short time). But things turn out okay.

The first time I tried drugs I was 14. The funny thing about it is that I wasn't trying to get high; I was attempting suicide. I took a whole bottle of Valium that I stole from my mother's medicine cabinet, and everything felt fine. I didn't die, and in fact for the first time in my life I had no fear, no anger, no anxiety, no sense of being overwhelmed or feelings of hopelessness, no despair – I felt nothing but a drug-induced euphoria and floated on that wave of pleasure all night long. It wasn't just that all those negative unpleasant feelings that had always been with me were gone – I actually felt good! From that moment on until I made it into recovery about 4½ years ago I would ingest (drink, snort, smoke, pop, shoot up, inhale) any and all substances that I thought would help me change the way I was feeling. And on that particular night that I'd taken Valium for the first time I'd been so angry and felt so overwhelmed that for me the only thing that made sense at the time was suicide. That feeling didn't change for a very long time.

Before I discovered at age 14 the blissful noxious escape that drugs could provide, I had already experienced what I guess is a fair bit of trauma. There'd been sexual abuse before age 6, physical abuse, emotional abuse, I'd also witnessed some really freaky scenes that shook me to the core and eroded any sense of safety I had faster than Hurricane Sandy demolished the Jersey Shore. I grew up in a beautiful, upper-middle-class town in northern New Jersey being raised by two highly educated parents until age 13, when they got a divorce. But I was "okay" – I didn't know that the abuse was abuse, and I just assumed my "crazy" thinking was because I was defective. I didn't know there were very real reasons why I felt so bad, hopeless, and afraid most of the time. What I did know was that I wasn't normal. I knew I didn't fit in anywhere, and I knew I'd never really be good at anything, and I knew if I did succeed at anything it was probably because it was easy or because the people I was competing against must really suck, and I knew nobody could really ever love me or want me in their lives, and I absolutely knew if anyone was nice to me it meant they wanted something from me. More sexual abuse began when I was 15, perpetrated by a "family friend," and from that point on I absolutely knew that if someone was nice to me it meant they wanted something sexual from me (and I also knew I could never, never, never say "no"). I knew I had a lot of friends, and I knew most of the time I didn't feel close to or connected with any of them. I knew I hated myself. I knew I felt numb a lot of the time and that the numbness slowly grew and carved through me like some glacier shaping my behaviors over my lifetime – so slowly, though, that I wasn't even aware it was happening. I knew suicide was something I'd considered young, even before 14, and was an option that I tragically carried with me for more than 25 years and that led to many near-lethal attempts, the most severe of which was at age 18, which left me blind, unable to walk, talk, and so cognitively impaired that I couldn't add 1 + 1.

My drinking escalated throughout high school, and I'd try anything that I could get my hands on that I believed would help me change the way I felt. During high school I mostly had access to alcohol, various pills (benzos and painkillers), and occasionally smoked marijuana as well as abused inhalants. I loved the feeling drugs and alcohol gave me – the soft white glow of a drug-induced high became my obsession. I only felt okay when I was under the influence. During high school I'd also had several overdoses resulting from suicide attempts that I hid from my family and friends.

I felt utterly alone. At my core was this belief that everyone was better than me and I was filled with shame and fear and embarrassment at the abuse that continued throughout high school and beyond. I was trapped, and it was all my fault. I really believed what I was experiencing was completely my fault. I didn't know how to safely ask for help, and my behaviors became riskier and riskier, and as a result I experienced many trips to the emergency room resulting from car crashes, fights, drug overdoses, and suicide attempts. When I was feeling anything it was pain, but I could never cry. And I wanted somebody to see me, to see the incredible pain I was in, but I was a shy, quiet kid from a good town and a good family, and that meant everything was okay.

My drug use and drinking escalated during college when I began using cocaine, and so did my trauma experience. I'd drive into Harlem and the Lower West Side of New York City, and also to very dangerous parts of Newark, New Jersey, to buy drugs. As a result of this I experienced gun violence, physical assaults, and also witnessed several horrific events, including one homicide. My sense of safety gone, my behavior reckless, flashbacks, dissociative episodes, depression, suicide attempts my norm, I sought out many psych hospitalizations and drug treatment centers hoping to recover. I might stay "well" for a day to several months (and at one time almost 1½ years) but was unable to build any foundation upon which a stable life could stand. Maybe I'd be sober, but bingeing and purging. Or sober, but cutting and looking at porn all the time. When I wasn't sober, though, all bets were off and the anger I felt toward myself and the world fueled binges of destruction so devastating that on the other side of them I'd swear I was done for good and head back to therapy, or AA, or a drug treatment center, or a psych hospital.

I was also unable to maintain long-term romantic relationships, and although in college I had a girlfriend for close to 3 years, I'd gotten to the point where 3 months seemed a long time for my relationships. I mean, this isn't really surprising – an unemployed, drug-addicted alcoholic living on Social Security disability who experiences severe dissociative episodes isn't like the best catch out there, but I'd tell myself I still looked pretty good, and for the year I was abusing steroids, I probably did.

I had been trying for so long (for my entire life) to show the world I was doing okay and convince myself the same, and finally I just gave up and stayed alone with my addictions and trauma reenactments for close to 5 years. That was the darkest period of my life. The despair I felt during those years was absolute, and when I wasn't drinking or drugging I was contemplating suicide. I felt hollow. I had been consumed by my trauma and addictions – all joy, happiness, hope, and energy to try had been gradually pushed from me by that glacier. I blamed myself for being weak-willed and for giving up on life. At the very end I decimated myself with methamphetamines, torturing my body and mind with instruments of pain that resembled the lewd outrage that was my abuse. For days on end with no sleep or food and only enough water to keep the sessions going, I'd relive my trauma because I needed the pain to take me ultimately to pleasure. I'd keep myself in a state of chemically induced homeostasis until the tension overwhelmed me and I'd have a break. I desperately wanted to get back what had been ripped from me. For the briefest of moments, after days of no sleep and drugs and reenactments, I'd have a sliver of peace. I'd be calm; there'd be a glimmer in the heavy stillness of my soul, and I'd say to myself, "See, things aren't so bad," and I'd feel cleansed and pure, and then the feeling would pass, and I'd have to begin the process of getting high all over again, because I absolutely could not face any semblance of the truth about myself. I'd learned long before to be a chameleon in order to survive, and so now I had no idea who the fuck I was anyway, except that I wasn't good.

So that's my experience with trauma and addictions. I am happy to tell you that Recovery is possible for anyone. I live a full, happy life today. I got married about a year ago. I've been sober over 5 years and have worked full-time at the same job for well over 3 years now. I have friends whom I feel connected to and, happily, I can cry when I feel pain, and life certainly comes with pain. But I also feel joy and happiness and can treat myself and others with kindness and compassion. I have a growing clarity about who I am, and I love who I am today, imperfect man that I am. What worked for me probably wouldn't work for everyone, which I think is fine because my Recovery is just that – *my* Recovery. But I am far from unique and found that a combination of cognitive-behavioral therapy skills, Seeking Safety, individual therapy, AA, huge amounts of compassion, a commitment to life, and a strong desire to change after my "Oh shit, I really do hate myself, but it looks like I'm not going to kill myself (ever), and that means I'm stuck here, so I better fucking change" moment brought me to my knees and had me asking the Universe for help. I cultivate that spiritual connection on a daily basis through practicing Qigong, praying, and trying to be of service to people. And I am going to be okay. So are you. It is difficult for people who haven't experienced trauma and addiction to fully grasp how incredibly tenuous life can seem and how incredibly difficult change is to sustain, but you're most certainly not alone (although it might feel that way). There is hope, and Recovery is possible (for anyone).

✧ What do you find most inspiring about David's story?

✧ What parts of his story are meaningful to you?

✧ What would you tell him if you could?

✧ Do you believe recovery is possible for anyone – including you?

4

It's medical – you're not crazy, lazy, or bad

... it's a healthy thing now and then to hang a question mark on the things you have long taken for granted.
—BERTRAND RUSSELL, 20th-century British philosopher

Hidden Problems

Trauma and addiction are incredibly common, yet often the most hidden of issues. This occurs among people, such as the family that does not see the trauma or addiction in their midst, and within people – the person who denies the reality of trauma or addiction despite clear evidence, such as lost jobs or relationships. You may have shame, guilt, or denial and may feel there are few, if any, people you can open up to about what's really going on. Even in some treatment programs, you may never be asked about both trauma and addiction.

✧ Do any of the following statements feel familiar to you?

Trauma

» "I just won't think about it."
» "I look strong, but inside I'm in pain."
» "In my family, no one talked about what was going on."
» "Maybe it wasn't all that bad."
» "If people really knew me, they would reject me."
» "I never told anyone what happened."
» "I'm so ashamed."

23

Addiction

» "I do it a lot more than anyone knows (gambling/sex/shopping/drugs)."
» "If people stopped hassling me about my drinking, I wouldn't have to hide it."
» "I can quit tomorrow."
» "It's other people's fault that I use."
» "My addiction isn't hurting anyone."
» "Sure I drink a lot, but so does everyone around me."
» "If you lived through what I lived through, you'd get high too."

New Understanding

Only recently have trauma and addiction problems come to be seen as medical disorders and, importantly, understood in relation to each other. Decades ago, both topics were largely hidden, and they still are in some places. They were swept under the rug, not discussed. Institutions, communities, and even treatment programs typically ignored them. It's major progress that these topics are now brought to light.

Addiction and trauma relate to specific medical conditions. These are just as important to identify as physical illnesses such as diabetes or cancer. You can come to see that you're not "crazy," but instead have medical conditions that need help. Addiction and trauma problems have biological roots, and various forms of help, including counseling, medication, and peer supports, are available for them.

Seeing them as medical issues – not a personal failure – matters. You may believe you're weak, not trying hard enough, or not good enough. Or as a defense against such feelings, you may believe the opposite – you're fine and everyone else is the problem when they give you feedback about your behavior. You may want to get better but keep finding yourself stuck: "One step forward, two steps back." Others may also blame you for your problems if they don't understand trauma and addiction. You do play a role, but often not as much or in the ways that you think. Recovery will take effort, but it's about directing your efforts based on accurate medical knowledge.

Trauma

"Driving home one night, she was sitting at a red light and found herself confronted by an armed drug addict, who forced his way into her car. . . . 'For eight months at least,' she said, 'every night before I went to bed, I'd think about it. I wouldn't be

able to sleep, so I'd get up, make myself a cup of decaf tea, watch something silly on TV to get myself out of that mood. And every morning I'd wake up feeling like I had a gun against my head.'"
—From "The Quest to Forget" (*New York Times*, 2004)

"I remember the exact moment when I decided to forget – I was six and I said, 'My grandfather is a good person who wouldn't hurt me. I must be making this up. I decided it was me, not him, that was the problem.'"
—Child abuse survivor

"When you survive a life-threatening experience you become a new person just like that. . . . I knew that I would make a full recovery physically, but I now lived in a world of medical mistakes, the body's betrayal, and life-threatening surprises. The present no longer felt safe."
—Michele Rosenthal, *Before the World Intruded: Conquering the Past and Creating the Future, A Memoir*

Trauma awareness is now stronger than ever before. There's recognition of all sorts of traumas, including child abuse, terrorism, war, violence, military stress, industrial accidents, and natural disasters such as hurricanes. Sex abuse scandals in institutions such as sports teams, the church, the military, and criminal justice settings have drawn attention to these previously hidden tragedies. Trauma is now recognized as happening to all ages, genders, and ethnicities. In earlier eras it was identified only in relation to men coming back from war, with terms such as *shell shock, combat stress reaction,* and *combat fatigue.*

"A Normal Reaction to Abnormal Events"

Trauma can have direct and sometimes lasting impact on how you feel. Problems from trauma include:

» Depression or sadness

» Flashbacks (unable to get trauma images out of your mind)

» Difficulty trusting others

» Fear of being attacked even when there's no actual threat

» Anger

» Trouble focusing on work or tasks

» Nightmares

» Relationship problems

» Spaciness

» Physical problems that your doctor can't explain, such as heart racing or nausea

» Panic or intense nervousness

» Impulses to hurt yourself or others

» Wanting to die

» Chronic pain

» Paranoia

» Hopelessness, giving up

» Shame, guilt

» Difficulty remembering parts of the trauma

» Avoiding reminders of the trauma

» Thoughts about the trauma that you can't get out of your mind

» Dissociation, which means the mind shuts down in response to stress

If you do have trauma problems, it's key to identify them without shame or blame. In earlier times and, sadly, sometimes still today, people with trauma problems were viewed as weak. There's now greater understanding that emotional distress makes sense after trauma – it's sometimes called "a normal reaction to abnormal events." You're not wrong or weak. You're not crazy.

Some people have ongoing problems from trauma, while others don't. Many people feel distress during or after trauma, but if the trauma was not severe, they usually feel better within 1 to 3 months. But this depends on the context:

o *How serious the trauma was.* More forceful traumas lead to worse distress. Being raped or assaulted usually has more intense emotional impact than witnessing a street fight, for example, although both can be traumas.

o *How others responded.* Was support available during or after trauma? Some people get compassionate care from their family, community, or professional helpers. Others are isolated, blamed, or shamed.

o *How well you were doing before the trauma.* If you were already having a hard time before the trauma, it may feel more devastating than if you felt strong and happy beforehand.

   o *Your family history.* If you have addiction or mental illness in your family, you're more likely to develop trauma and addiction problems. Culture can also play a role (see "Every child is a detective," Chapter 22).

Even the same trauma can have a different impact on different people. Imagine two people who survive a car accident: one emerges shaken but just happy to be alive with no lasting problems; the other can't get over it even months later.

   Whatever your reactions to trauma, you can get better.

Medical Conditions

Several medical conditions directly relate to trauma:

   o *Acute stress disorder*: immediate, major distress that lasts up to a month after a trauma.

   o *Posttraumatic stress disorder* (PTSD): emotional distress from trauma that lasts for more than a month and sometimes for years. About 20% of people who suffer trauma develop PTSD. But among people who had severe trauma, such as rape, sexual abuse, violent assault, and mass violence, 60–80% develop PTSD.

   o *Adjustment disorder*: difficulty coping with a stressful event, which may show up as depressed mood, anxiety, and behavior problems. Adjustment disorders usually heal quickly.

   o *Complex trauma reactions*: This is a widely used term, but is not a formal medical condition. It's sometimes called *complex PTSD,* and it refers to problems that may develop in people who lived through ongoing trauma such as child abuse, domestic violence, or torture. These experiences derail normal development, leading to lack of a strong sense of self, feeling fragmented, difficulty forming healthy relationships, physical harm to self or others, medical problems, memory problems, intense and unstable feelings, and doubting of one's own perceptions.

   o *Dissociative identity disorder*: This used to be called *multiple personality disorder.* Although very rare, it can arise from extreme, repeated, severe childhood trauma. The person has major memory gaps and an identity that is fragmented into different "alters" (personalities), who may be different ages and genders and may not be aware of each other.

Note: In children, trauma problems may be expressed in play rather than in words. For children under age 6, there are different criteria to identify PTSD. See "Resources" (Appendix B) to learn more about that and other topics related to trauma.

✳ Explore . . . *Do you have trauma problems?*

If you're unsure whether you have trauma problems, try any of these options.

- *Take a screening test.* Answer a set of free, brief, anonymous questions privately on your own. See "Resources" (Appendix B) for how to find such tests.

- *Obtain a formal evaluation by a professional.* Be sure to find someone who has training in trauma and uses valid measures for assessing trauma problems.

- *Read more about trauma.* Keep reading here and elsewhere. Sometimes just listening to yourself with an open heart can help you figure out where you're at and what you need. See "Resources" (Appendix B) for good websites and books.

Addiction

"Addiction was a 'forest fire that burned through everything in its path and left only charred remains'; it began with cough syrup and ended with heroin and alcohol."
—Chuck Negron, from *The Harder They Fall: Celebrities Tell Their Real-Life Stories of Addiction and Recovery*

"I would say, 'I need wine for that recipe,' and really believed that's why I was buying it."
—Karin, a homemaker and alcoholic

"Gambling gives me a big adrenaline rush, like what I used to get in combat. I need that high. Civilian life is boring, like a black-and-white movie instead of color."
—Luis, a military veteran

"It's about passion, sensual pleasure, deep pulls, lust, fears, yearning hungers. It's about needs so strong they're crippling."
—Carolyn Knapp, from *Drinking: A Love Story*

People can become addicted to anything that gives pleasure or relief. Everyone wants to enjoy life, but if you can't put the brakes on a behavior or it's causing problems, it's time to look at it carefully. Addiction is a real illness – it's not about just wanting to have a good time or lack of willpower. In earlier times it was viewed as weakness and even as possession by the devil, but now it's understood to have biological and social causes ("nature and nurture"). There's also more understanding of behavioral addictions such as gambling, sex, food, and shopping.

In general you may notice an addiction problem based on:

» *Quantity*: too much of a behavior.

» *Loss of control*: feeling that you can't stop even if you want to.

» *The toll it takes on your life*: major financial, medical, emotional, legal, family, or social problems.

» *Feedback from others*: they may notice a problem before you do.

» *Impulsiveness*: you are repeatedly triggered to do it.

You may already know that you have an addiction but wonder whether you have other ones. Or you may question whether you have any addiction at all. Or maybe you notice a few problems and aren't sure whether you're at risk for developing a full-blown addiction. Later in this chapter you can answer some questions to better understand your own situation.

Addiction Problems Can Be Mild, Moderate, or Severe

You may think it's not an addiction unless you're falling-down drunk, homeless, a criminal, unemployed, or overdosing. But you may have a problem even if no one notices it or you don't yet see it in yourself, even if you're successful in other areas of your life, even if you're a kind and decent person, and even if you take good care of yourself overall. In fact people who look good to others are the least likely to be noticed as having an addiction problem, such as successful parents, professionals, and good students. Some are called *functioning addicts* – they function well at work and home even while being addicted.

Addiction problems can be *mild, moderate,* or *severe.* It's best to catch addiction as early as possible to prevent it from getting worse – "hear the whisper before it becomes a scream." Rethinking Drinking, for example, is a free government website to help prevent people who have a mild drinking problem from becoming full-blown alcoholics. You can work to reduce *problem gambling,* the mild version, so that it doesn't become *gambling disorder*, the severe version. See "Resources" (Appendix B) for more on these.

You may have a mild addiction *heading down* (in early stages of addiction) or *coming back up* (as you recover from a full-blown addiction). Wherever you're at, be honest about your problems so that you can tell whether you're getting better or worse over time.

Yet no matter how severe an addiction is, it's never too late for recovery. See "'Things turn out okay' – David's experience" (Chapter 3) for a real-life example of someone with severe addictions who has had lasting recovery.

Many Types of Addiction

Substance Addictions

Substance addiction is common and is what most people think of when they hear the word *addiction*. There are many different substances, and the list keeps growing as new ones emerge. Alcohol has been around through most of human history, but most abused drugs are modern inventions that arose as chemists started developing them from the mid-1800s on, with cocaine, heroin, and opiates becoming popular during the late 1800s.

Alcohol is the most common substance addiction in part because it's the only one that's legal in most places as a recreational substance. Marijuana is the most commonly used illegal drug, and with legalization of marijuana increasing, addiction to it is on the rise. Aside from which substances are legal, it's clear that different drugs wax and wane in popularity. Cocaine was big in the 1890s and also in the 1980s. Marijuana was big in the 1970s, went down in the 1990s, and is now back up again.

Even though there are many different names for substances that can be abused, they boil down to four basic types: *opioids* (such as heroin and OxyContin); *stimulants* (such as cocaine, Ecstasy, speed, and methamphetamine); *hallucinogens* (such as LSD, peyote, and hallucinogenic mushrooms); *depressants* (such as alcohol, Valium, and Seconal); and some that are a mix (such as marijuana).

Behavioral Addictions

There are also *behavioral addictions*, although most are not yet formally recognized in the medical field. Gambling addiction is the most studied and is recognized as a medical problem. Other possible behavioral addictions that are currently being studied include shopping or spending, sex, pornography, electronics (such as Internet, texting, gaming, television), work, exercise, and hobbies. There are also reports of less common behavioral addictions such as tanning, plastic surgery, tattooing, and visiting psychics. Eating is sometimes considered a behavioral addiction, but in medical terms it's called *binge-eating disorder,* or, if there's purging after the binge, such as vomiting, it's called *bulimia.*

Although behavioral addictions have been studied less than substance addictions, they are being recognized more and more. They appear to evoke the same brain changes as substance addiction, although more studies are needed on this. They are also experienced similarly, including craving, difficulty stopping, guilt, shame, and compulsive repetition of the behavior. (See "Excessive Behavior Scale," Appendix C.)

Signs of an Addiction Problem

The quiz below offers a list of questions to help you figure out if you have an addiction. You don't have to say "yes" to all of them to have a problem. And remember that you don't have to use the word *addiction* if you prefer some other term such as *issue, problem,* or *addictive behavior.*

> ✧ As you read each question, try to really notice, without judgment or blame, if it feels true for you. You can answer the questions for a substance, such as alcohol or drugs, or they can be applied to behavior, such as gambling, Internet use, sex, work, gaming, and so on. Go through the list more than once if you have more than one behavior that may be a problem.

Do you . . .

1. Continue to do it even when it causes relationship problems?	Yes / Maybe / No
2. Want to cut down but aren't able to?	Yes / Maybe / No
3. Have cravings and urges to do it?	Yes / Maybe / No
4. Do it more or longer than you intend to?	Yes / Maybe / No
5. Spend a lot of time getting, doing, or recovering from it?	Yes / Maybe / No
6. Not manage what you should be doing at work, home, or school because of it?	Yes / Maybe / No

7. Give up important social, work, or leisure activities because of it?   Yes / Maybe / No

8. Do it again and again even when it puts you in danger?   Yes / Maybe / No

9. Continue to do it even though you know you have a physical or   Yes / Maybe / No
   emotional problem that gets worse from it?

10. Need to do more of it to get the effect you want (*tolerance*)?   Yes / Maybe / No

11. Have withdrawal symptoms (nervousness, irritation, headaches,   Yes / Maybe / No
    depression, sweating, heart racing, or tension) when you don't do
    it for a while, and then these go away when you return to it?

> ✧ How many questions did you answer with "yes" or "maybe"? Your problem
> is likely *mild* if you said "yes" or "maybe" to just two or three of the
> questions; *moderate* if four or five; and *severe* if six or more. To find out for
> sure, see the next section.

✳ Explore . . . *Do you have an addiction problem?*

If you're unclear whether you have addiction problems, try any of these options.

- *Take a screening test.* Answer a set of free, brief, anonymous questions privately on your own. You can take screening tests for alcohol, drugs, and
  behavioral addictions. See "Resources" (Appendix B) to find such tests.

- *Obtain a formal evaluation from a professional.* Be sure to find someone who
  has training in addiction and uses valid measures for it.

- *Read more about addiction.* See "Resources" (Appendix B) for websites and
  books. Sometimes just listening closely can help you figure out the truth
  about yourself.

Addiction can be tricky to figure out. It may be hard to accurately see a problem, as
denial is part of the illness. The field of mental health has also had different definitions over time and recognizes some addictions more than others. Most behavioral
addictions are not yet formally recognized by professionals. But grassroots 12-step
groups exist for gambling, work, sex, eating, and spending addictions, for example.
Twelve-step groups refers to the most widespread addiction recovery model, which
began with Alcoholics Anonymous in 1935 and later expanded to other addictions.
Knowledge continues to evolve, so seek as much information as you can.

"An Octopus": Trauma and Addiction Touch Many Other Life Problems

Trauma and addiction are only part of the story; both are linked to other problems too. They're like an octopus – reaching out and touching many aspects of your life.

✧ Notice any problems below that are present in your life.

> » *Social problems* such as isolation, loneliness, and not getting along with others.
> » *Anger problems*: too much or too little anger.
> » *Financial problems.*
> » *Physical health problems.*
> » *Difficulty with tasks,* such as keeping a job and taking care of children.
> » *Legal problems,* such as driving-under-the-influence (DUI) arrests, loss of custody of children, drug charges, and other criminal activity.
> » *Risk of HIV and AIDS.*
> » *Harm to self or others,* such as suicidal or violent impulses.
> » *Homelessness.*
> » *Domestic violence.*

Many people have such problems, but never link them to trauma and addiction. Seeing those connections may help you take a more compassionate view of yourself and others, especially if you have severe trauma or addiction problems.

Recovery Is Possible

If you've struggled for a long time with trauma and addiction, you may feel hopeless about getting better: "Nothing will work." "I'm not strong enough." "I've used for so long, I can't stop." You may have gone through treatment yet still have problems. But recovery from both trauma and addiction *is* possible. Medical research shows that both can improve even if you had them for years. Most people never receive help designed for both trauma and addiction at the same time. The idea is not just *more* help but *different* help.

✧ How does it feel to view trauma problems as a medical issue?

✧ How does it feel to view addiction as a medical issue?

RECOVERY VOICES

Jasmin – "Part of the human race"

"I remember when I first found out I had PTSD. I was in treatment for cocaine addiction, and my counselor figured it out after we talked about the abuse that went on in my childhood. She pointed out to me that I had PTSD, not just a cocaine problem. At first I was like, 'Oh, you're kidding, I can't have all these conditions at one time.' But then I was relieved to know that I had something with a name. For so long I thought there was just something wrong with me – no cure for this. But I can deal with it now. It's different when you don't know. But when you find out, it's like people with cancer: they find out where their sickness comes from, and they can work on it. This chapter reminds me how I saw myself so differently after I understood all that – like I'm part of the human race now, even if I'm a person with these problems. Before that I always felt so ashamed, so freakish, like I couldn't do anything right. This has me feeling hopeful – I know what I need to work on."

5

How do people change?

This time, like all times, is a very good one, if we but know what to do with it.

—RALPH WALDO EMERSON, 19th-century American writer

There are so many different types of counseling, self-help, medications, and spiritual methods that it can get confusing to answer the essential question: How do people change?

This chapter offers a wide-angle view of how change happens, focusing on eight core ways. Although there are different brand names for change methods, all of them are basically rooted in one or more of these key processes.

✧ Mark which of the eight methods appeal to you most.

1. Learning New Coping

Coping refers to how you respond to problems. In healthy families and communities, good coping is part of the "air you breathe" – it's shown in action by people around you even if they don't talk about it. They are responsible, and they manage challenges in positive ways. But trauma and addiction reduce your ability to cope, sometimes dramatically. You may need to learn or relearn the "how to's" of life: how to calm

---

This chapter was adapted with permission from *Creating Change* by Lisa M. Najavits (forthcoming from The Guilford Press).

yourself when upset . . . manage triggers . . . rethink situations . . . set boundaries in relationships . . . take better care of your body . . . feel pleasure without addictive behavior, and so on. See "Safe coping skills" (Chapter 12) for more.

What Learning New Coping Feels Like

Dylan was 28 when he found out he had Hodgkin's disease. He had used alcohol and marijuana several times a week since he was 15. "The cancer shook up everything. I was a work-hard, party-hard guy. When the doctor told me I'd have to give up the drinking and weed, that hit me harder than the idea of going through chemo. I told myself I didn't have an addiction because I could hold down a job. But when I tried to stop, it scared me that I couldn't stick to it. So I went to rehab. The main therapy, in addition to AA, was coping skills – hour after hour of the stuff: anger management, mood management, cognitive-behavioral skills, relapse prevention skills. It was like a master's degree in coping. At first I was like, 'This won't work when I'm back home.' But I kept coming back to the words *cancer* and *death* and knew I had to try. I was surprised the skills helped me. It was life-hacker stuff: how to handle cravings, how to deal with people, how to have fun without partying. It wasn't easy, but I finally got that I have the power to decide how to act in any given situation whether it's cravings or getting pissed at someone or anything else. I would never have wished for cancer, but I'm grateful for what I learned. I got through the cancer treatment and have been clean from substances for 2 years now."

✧ Are there any new coping skills you want to learn?

2. Grieving

Trauma and losses can be grieved. You can let yourself feel the emotional pain, moving through it and emerging with new understanding and a sense of peace. You can't change the events of the past, but you can change how you feel about them. Grieving is especially helpful for losses – loss of time, physical health, innocence. It can also help you come to terms with what should have been present but wasn't, such as love and compassion. If trauma or addiction are severe, it may feel like your entire life went off track; this too can be grieved. You may have also lost people and places that you loved. If you decide to do grief work, be sure to see "Two types of trauma counseling" (Chapter 33), as grieving can be emotionally overwhelming. It can set off addiction relapse if you're not ready for it and if you don't do it carefully.

What Grieving Feels Like

The writer Anne Lamott, who has written openly about her trauma and addiction, describes grieving: "[A]fter my dad died . . . I had to shut down almost entirely and just lie in the mud for months. I felt that the world was no longer safe if my young handsome lively father could be so suddenly dead. It felt like it was a shooting gallery out there. And I felt like my heart had been so thoroughly and irreparably broken that there could be no real joy again, that at best there might eventually be a little contentment. Everyone wanted me to get help and rejoin life, pick up the pieces and move on, and I tried to, I wanted to, but I just had to lie in the mud with my arms wrapped around myself, eyes closed, grieving, until I didn't have to anymore. And then over time I became more or less okay: I did feel joy again, and I feel it now sometimes bigger than I ever thought possible. It's so big inside me . . . it's like a secret that might make me burst, like when you're in love."
—From *Operating Instructions*

✧ Would grieving losses help your recovery? If so, how can you do it carefully?

✧ Would it help to have the support of a counselor, group, or safe friend?

3. Quantum Change (Conversion)

Quantum change, also called *conversion,* is a sudden, dramatic, and permanent change. It's sometimes called "seeing the light" or "a bolt from the blue." It's different from the more common slow and steady recovery that has ups and downs along the way (which is referred to as *educational* or *incremental* change). In contrast, quantum change is "sudden, unplanned, profound, positive, and permanent – a recovery conversion experience [is one] in which one's life is forever cleaved into the categories of 'before' and 'after' in a matter of moments," according to addiction recovery writer William White. In addiction, *hitting bottom* sometimes results in quantum change. Losing a job, going to jail, getting into a car accident, or any other major addiction consequence can get a person to finally see that an addiction is out of control and unmanageable, which sparks permanent abstinence from substances. It's also called *the point of despair.* Quantum change often has a spiritual component and is described as being reborn: " . . . addictions were embedded within a damaged self that had to die before a new self could be born" (White, 2014). It's most often described in relation to addiction recovery rather than trauma.*

What Quantum Change (Conversion) Feels Like

A historic description of conversion comes from William James's 1902 book, *Varieties of Religious Experience*. Indeed, AA was developed based on James's descriptions of conversion experiences in that book – so much so that Bill Wilson, a founder of AA, said James should be considered a co-founder. The description here is religious in nature, but conversion can also occur in nonreligious contexts: "One Tuesday evening I sat in a saloon in Harlem, a homeless, friendless, dying drunkard. I had pawned or sold anything that would bring a drink. I could not sleep unless I was dead drunk. I had not eaten for days . . . it came into my head to go to Jerry M'Auley's Mission . . . I listened to the testimony of twenty-five or thirty persons, every one of whom had been saved from rum, and I made up my mind that I would be saved or die right there . . . I knelt down with a crowd of drunkards . . . and then, with a breaking heart, I said, 'Dear Jesus, can you help me?' Never with a mortal tongue can I describe that moment. Although up to that moment my soul had been filled with indescribable gloom, I felt the glorious brightness of the noonday sun into my heart. I felt I was a free man. . . . From that moment on until now I have never wanted a drink of whiskey."

⟡ Do you want to learn more about quantum change? Talk to people at 12-step meetings; read *The Big Book of AA*. There is also a self-help book called *Quantum Change*. (See References.)

4. Relationship-Based Change

Loving relationships can be one of the most powerful methods of change. The relationships may be with family, friends, a counselor, a spiritual source such as a higher power, or a self-help group. Caring relationships are especially important in recovery from trauma and addiction, as these erode healthy connections with others. Trauma

---

*In the PTSD field, *conversion* has the opposite meaning of that in the addiction field. PTSD conversion refers to someone becoming ill rather than becoming well. A person suffers extreme trauma, represses it (does not acknowledge the trauma or feelings it evokes), and as a result becomes physically incapacitated such as going blind, deaf, or becoming paralyzed. There are various reports of such conversions, including among military personnel during World War I as well as in modern times.

can make it hard for you to trust others, and addiction can make it hard for others to trust you, for example. Your recovery can also be strengthened in relationships in which you help others such as being a parent, an AA sponsor, or a peer helping other trauma survivors.

What Relationship-Based Change Feels Like

Cassie lost her parents when she was 7 and grew up in a foster family where there was neglect and abuse. She developed an alcohol problem as an adult when her own daughter turned 7, which brought up painful memories for her. "My husband sat down and talked with me. I was drinking too much. I was driving while drunk. He loves me dearly and was concerned for my safety. I was able to hear him, and I entered AA. When I look back on what I was like 8 months ago when I started AA and became sober versus now, I'm amazed at the changes. In the beginning, I felt like I would never make it – but one meeting at a time, working the steps, turning to my sponsor – has brought me through a storm of emotions and doubt and fear to this more secure place. I can trust myself a little more and feel more able to handle my emotions. I know this is still considered the beginning of recovery, and I wonder what I will feel like at my first anniversary, in 5 years, and in 10 years. I also now know that I need support around my childhood trauma. As I learn more about it, I see why I began drinking. I'm in awe of my husband's love and how he told me the truth of what he was seeing in a way that got me to change."

✧ Do you have relationships that help your recovery? If not, is there one you could begin to build?

5. Physically Based Change

This type of change occurs through medication, body therapies, or other strong physical experiences. There's growing awareness that mind–body connections promote healing, and for some people the physical realm is more compelling than traditional verbal help such as counseling. Trauma and addiction problems may be helped through physical methods such as yoga, exercise, massage, and qigong. Psychiatric medications are one of the most common physical change methods for trauma problems (e.g., antidepressants) as well as for addiction (to reduce cravings, to substitute for opiates, etc.).

What Physically Based Change Feels Like

Michele had PTSD for over a decade from a severe, life-threatening physical illness at age 13. "[My therapist] explains that the brain encodes experience in neural pathways and that in the case of life-threatening experiences, those neural pathways can become overactive. Our goal is to 'process out' the experience of my illness. . . . We use information processing techniques: eye movement desensitization and reprocessing, thought field therapy, emotional freedom technique, and Tapas acupressure technique. . . . Little by little, the creaky machinery of the mind–body connection, which was shut down and boarded up so many years ago, begins to turn on a well-greased axis. I begin to recognize my instincts and where and how they reside in the reactions of my body. I begin to practice listening for and gauging the strength of that inner voice. . . . I train myself to feel impulse and respond, no questions asked. Soon, this sort of behavior becomes automatic, and I begin walking around feeling all warm and fuzzy with the thought that maybe, just maybe, there's a way to join back together my Before and After selves, my fear and my strength."

—From *Before the World Intruded: Conquering the Past and Creating the Future, A Memoir,* by Michele Rosenthal

---

✧ Would it help you to try some physical recovery methods?

6. Coercion

Coercion refers to forced change such as being legally required to attend treatment ("mandated"). It's used for addiction treatment but rarely, if ever, for trauma. It may surprise you to learn that people who are forced to attend treatment do just as well as or better than those who attend voluntarily, according to research. And some people say being forced into treatment was the best thing that ever happened to them. Psychiatrist Kathleen Brady describes how many people need a push, even if not always formal coercion, to get into treatment: "I haven't had one patient that came in because they woke up one day out of the clear blue and said, 'I'm an addict. And I need to get clean. . . . Generally, everybody has their arm twisted behind their back by something. They're either in trouble at work, their wife insists they come in, their kids have confronted them. It's the job of the treatment professionals to really hook them into treatment."

Renee's Story: What Coercion Feels Like

"I used to think a drug addict was someone who lived on the far edge of society, wild-eyed with a shaven head and living in filthy squalor. That was until I became one. You see, I never thought I was an addict. In my mind, I was functioning just fine, so I thought. I lived in a lovely home, drove a nice car, was a mom, a wife, and had a great career. I guess you could say I was living the American dream. That was until my addiction to prescription pain killers turned my life upside down. My addiction introduced me to the legal system and forced me into treatment. At the time, I thought it was a punishment, but in fact it saved my life! . . . Little by little, my walls of protection started to come down. My counselor helped me understand that emotional pain hurts just as much as, if not more than, physical pain. I never thought that I would be able to break through the pain and chain of addiction that was wrapped so tightly around me, but I did. . . . Today I am in recovery from this life-threatening disease. I feel happy, joyous, and free, am a better wife and mother . . . and am preparing for a new career as an addictions counselor to be of service to others."

✧ Do you need a push to get into recovery? How could that push happen?

7. Consequences

"Everybody, sooner or later, sits down to a banquet of consequences," the writer Robert Louis Stevenson said. Some consequences feel good, such as praise, applause, or an A in school. Some consequences feel bad, such as being scolded or getting into debt. There are also formal methods for consequences such as an *intervention,* in which family and friends organize to confront a person about addiction ("No more financial support until you enter treatment"). Getting an AA chip is a consequence. Drug urine testing is tied to various consequences. But consequences in life aren't always clear. You may get rejected by people and not know why. Consequences can also be unfair, such as when you're discriminated against or denied opportunities that you deserve. Trauma and addiction result in all sorts of consequences – some fair, some unfair. People who do best in recovery pay attention to consequences. They observe the impact of their behavior and try to stay on the good side of consequences as much as possible. They hear the feedback life is offering.

What Consequences Feel Like

Anna was addicted to cybersex: "Once I got online I suddenly had access to the biggest singles bar in the world. . . . In the digital world it was easy to approach people I was interested in and to walk away from those I wasn't interested in. . . . The problem was that I forgot about my real life. The allure and the excitement of online romances were just stronger than my need to go to work, pay rent, buy groceries, and take care of myself. Over time, my life gradually fell apart until I was completely alone and desperate. Eventually my siblings stepped in. . . . I'm so glad they did. Now I have a job that I like, and a nice apartment, and I've even started dating. I haven't met the right guy for me, but that's okay. I'm probably not ready for a serious romance anyway. But someday I will be, thanks to my recovery."
—From *Always Turned On: Sex Addiction in the Digital Age,* by Robert Weiss and Jennifer P. Schneider

---

✧ What consequences can promote a stronger recovery for you?

8. Creativity

Creativity and healing are directly related. Creativity helps you access parts of yourself you can't access otherwise. It allows you to convert emotional pain into authentic expressions of your truth that inspire others or contribute to the world. Creativity can occur through traditional arts such as painting, writing, and theater; and broadly, through intellectual work, spiritual pursuit, or a social justice mission. It can occur by engaging in others' creative work such as going to galleries and concerts. All of these open up your inner world and let you play with possibilities through different perspectives and ways of expression.

What Creativity Feels Like

A woman who survived child abuse and alcoholism said, "Art became a wonderful release. It's like I could go from all the trauma and all the craziness in my life over into this one area that was safe, where I could just express and be creative and do what I wanted to do. I could be totally in control of what was on that canvas. The

nude that I painted when I was 20 . . . I think the story behind her is that the female body is something of beauty and is to be appreciated and respected."
—From the video *Trauma: No More Secrets*

✧ What creative activities could help your recovery?

Try as Many Different Change Methods as You Can

The more ways you try, the better your chance of lasting change. You don't have to feel motivated, and you don't have to believe that any one specific way will work. You just have to show up, try what you can, and keep at it. Put one foot in front of the other over and over. Come up with a plan now. Give yourself a reasonable period of time, such as 2 months, and then notice whether you see any change. Make adjustments and keep going. Then give it another few months, and so on. Don't give up if something doesn't work; keep trying other ways.

Debbie struggles with food addiction and trauma memories. She uses many different methods of change: "I'm learning ways to cope with overwhelming feelings, with flashbacks, migraines, nightmares. I find that if I hum softly to myself, I can reduce the panic that arises inside of me. I find that if I cut back on too much work and activity and eat nutritiously, I'm able to manage my migraines. I am working with my psychopharm doctor and neurologist to find the right medications to help with all of my symptoms. I am working with a therapist to help with the PTSD and dissociation. I am starting to run and exercise regularly. I have begun to feel alive!"

Experiment with Different Formats

Each of the eight methods in this chapter is a core *process* of change, and each of them also comes in different *formats*. For example, if you're interested in the change process *learning new coping*, you could do that using any of these formats:

» Read about it.
» Go to counseling.
» Attend a class.

» Go to a self-help group.
» Observe how others do it.

◇ What methods of change may work for you?

◇ Who or what can help you launch new ways of changing? Online resources? A friend? A doctor or other professional?

RECOVERY VOICES

Curtis – "I became proud to be who I was."

"I was injured in 1968 in Vietnam during my military service. I lost the use of my hand and went through 12 operations at Walter Reed Army Hospital. I was a patient there for 18 months and then came home. Readjustment to civilian life was really hard. For the first 2 years I pretty much did what I had done in Vietnam. I was up all night and slept in the day. I was running around the streets and pretty much re-creating the trauma, dealing with a lot of unsavory people, hanging out in places where I shouldn't have been, and drinking and carrying on. How did I change? It was a mix of different things, a lot like what's described in this chapter. Grieving was part of it – letting myself feel the emotional pain, moving through it. I was able to do that by doing a long-term inpatient program early in my recovery. Luckily, too, when I was wandering through the wilderness I found AA, and it's been wonderful ever since. I've been sober for over 20 years. I've also been in treatments of various kinds to learn new coping and certainly had my share of consequences that life has dealt me. I'm very impressed with this chapter. It's one of my favorites in the book because we talk about change – but really, how do you change? It's something easy to say, but how do you actually do it? This chapter is a step-by-step recipe for how to change yourself. It's excellent. It helps take away the fear of change. When you start out, you have this fear – you're lying to yourself, afraid to face what's really going on, and not at all sure of what to do. For me, once I began really working on changing myself the fear went away. I became proud to be who I was. I'm a grateful recovering alcoholic."

6

The world is your school

All the world is my school and all humanity is my teacher.
—GEORGE WHITMAN, 20th-century American intellectual and recipient
   of the French Order of Arts and Letters

Be inspired by others. Various websites offer stories of recovery by those who lived it, in their own words. All of the following are nonprofit, free, reputable resources. You can find others by searching online for "personal stories" and a keyword such as "trauma," "PTSD," "addiction," "homelessness," or "domestic violence."

» **Military veterans in recovery from trauma, their family members and counselors**
   Videos
   www.ptsd.va.gov/apps/AboutFace

» **People with substance abuse, mental health issues, or both**
   Brief written accounts
   www.heretohelp.bc.ca/personal-stories

» **People with PTSD**
   Brief written accounts
   www.adaa.org/living-with-anxiety/personal-stories
   Videos
   www.pickingupthepeaces.org.au/ptsd-disorder/ptsd-symptoms/living-with-ptsd

» **People with addiction**
   Brief written accounts
   www.storiesofrecovery.org.uk/index.php

Videos
www.inexcess.tv

» **People with addiction and/or mental health problems**
Brief written accounts
www.recoverymonth.gov/personal-stories/read
www.ncadd.org/people-in-recovery/recovery-stories
Video
www.youtube.com/playlist?list=PLAWzAhT15N-qurIyzUG8bI8OHA1w80utI

» **Domestic violence survivors**
Video
www.upworthy.com/ever-tell-yourself-youre-in-love-with-a-deeply-difficult-person-instead-of-facing-the-truth

⬧ What do you find inspiring when you watch the videos?

⬧ Write down some words of wisdom you hear from people on the videos.

RECOVERY VOICES

Simone – "Turn your face toward the light."

"I really like working on this. I'm early in recovery from trauma and alcohol abuse, and it's helped me become more positive about that. It's not easy when you're stuck in the negative to frame it in a positive way for yourself, but once you can see how other people have done it you can hang on to it and reach for it. When I'm going through dark, difficult times, I remind myself of what someone said to me: 'The light is over there – all you have to do right in this moment is turn your face toward the light. That's all you have to do right now; nothing more. You don't have to walk toward it. Just turn toward it and you're doing your job.' And that's what recovery has been like for me so far. The only way I've been able to do it is with that baby step and then people start showing up to help, and I feel like maybe I'll get there. I'm still on the journey, but I'm getting there. It's a big life project for me. This chapter gives me a very clear way to keep turning toward the light. I get inspired by other people's recovery stories and then I feel like it may be possible for me."

7

Listen to your behavior

Honesty is the first chapter in the book of wisdom.
—THOMAS JEFFERSON, 18th-century statesman and American president

Watch Your Actions – More Than Your Feelings, Thoughts, or Words

As you go through your day you notice all sorts of things – feelings, people around you, tasks to do, the weather, colors in the room, noises, and much else. It's an ever-changing jumble of experiences in real time. It's "a blooming, buzzing confusion," as William James famously said.

But as you recover from trauma and addiction, it's important to prioritize one thing above all: your actions. Your behavior needs to become your compass. Trauma and addiction create a whirlwind of experiences that cloud your ability to see what's really happening. You may feel fine one moment and down the next.

Most people look to how they *feel* as a guide to how they're doing. But this is deceptive if you have addiction and trauma problems. You may feel bad but are doing fine – your mood is low but you're doing what you need to do, such as taking care of your kids and holding a job. Or it may be the opposite: you feel good but are doing poorly. You may be on the *pink cloud* – a fantasy of overconfidence and good feeling but perhaps heading toward relapse, rather than staying grounded in reality. By using your behavior as your one true guide you can stay centered and focus on what matters most.

Notice Whether Your Behaviors Are Safe or Unsafe

There are many behaviors to "listen to," but one key principle: notice whether they are safe or unsafe. You can also use other words:

47

» *Healthy* versus *unhealthy* behavior

» *Positive* versus *negative* behavior

» *Green light (go)* versus *red light (stop)*

✧ What words do you prefer?

Remember that this is about your behavior. It's not a judgment of you as a person. You may be doing the best you know, given your circumstances and what you learned from others. These are behaviors and choices, not praise or blame.

✭ Explore . . . *Is it safe or unsafe?*

Mark each item below as safe (S) or unsafe (U) or, if you're not sure, enter a question mark (?). The suggested answers are at the end of the chapter.

1. "When I'm depressed, I turn off the phone and sleep all day."   _____

2. "I go to the gym to get my mind off using."   _____

3. "I lie to my doctor because she wouldn't understand."   _____

4. "I'm already overweight, so I let myself have the doughnuts."   _____

5. "I limit gaming to an hour a day."   _____

6. "I don't go to events where there's drinking."   _____

7. "I hide how much I'm spending."   _____

8. "I let my 10-year-old daughter take care of herself when I go out."   _____

9. "Sometimes I don't go outside for days."   _____

10. "I set up a dentist appointment that I've been avoiding."   _____

11. "I threatened to kill a guy who disrespected me."   _____

12. "I get high and watch porn for hours."   _____

13. "I attend counseling."   _____

14. "I'm making a fruit salad instead of chocolate cake."   _____

15. "I use condoms if it might be unsafe sex."   _____

16. "When I wake up from nightmares, I cut myself."   _____

17. "I'm filling out an application to go back to school."   _____

18. "I went to a SMART Recovery meeting this week."   _____

19. "I hang out at bars to make new friends."   _____

20. "I signed up for parenting classes."   _____

21. "I'm getting a nicotine patch to get off cigarettes."   _____

How Can You Figure Out If Your Behavior Is Safe or Unsafe?

Most everyone has unsafe behavior at times, such as driving over the speed limit or eating or drinking too much. What makes it a problem is how often it happens, whether it's impulsive (indicating a lack of control), and whether it has a major or ongoing negative impact.

Also, what's safe or unsafe for you may not be for someone else. Working long hours at a job may be healthy for you but unsafe for a person with work addiction. Figuring out what is safe and unsafe for *you* requires eyes-wide-open honesty and feedback from people who know you well.

The general guidelines below may also help you evaluate your behavior.

Unsafe	Safe
Passive, drifting	Actively trying to improve
Yelling, fighting	Communicating calmly
Unproductive (not getting much done)	Productive (job, school, housework, etc.)
Spending time with people who drag you down, hurt you, or encourage addiction	Spending time with safe, supportive people
Letting responsibilities slip	Being responsible; taking care of what you need to
Physical harm to yourself or others	No physical harm
No planning; impulsive	Careful planning

<u>Unsafe</u>	<u>Safe</u>
Having fun in dangerous ways	Having fun in healthy ways
Taking unnecessary risks (e.g., driving drunk)	Protecting yourself from risks (e.g., calling a cab)
Dishonest	Honest
Addictive behavior	No addictive behavior

✦ In the past week, did you have more safe or unsafe behaviors?

✦ What are examples of each for you?

You Can Have Any Feelings at All – "Good, Bad, or Ugly" – as Long as Your Behaviors Are Safe

"I hate having feelings. Why does sobriety have to come with feelings? One minute I feel excited, the next I feel terrified. One minute I feel free and the next I feel doomed."
—From *Dry: A Memoir* by Augusten Burroughs

You can have all kinds of feelings: angry, sad, scared, vengeful, and anything else. Everyone has feelings like that, and trauma and addiction increase their intensity. But the feelings don't have to lead to unsafe behavior. They can just come and go. Telling yourself you shouldn't have them makes it harder, like having "thought police" inside of you – one more thing to feel bad about. So it's always your *behavior* that can keep you on track, that one essential question, that touchstone to return to: Is your behavior safe or unsafe? You may have safe behaviors with negative feelings. You may have unsafe behavior with positive feelings. It can all get confusing and jumbled. So keep coming back, like a dog to a bone, to that one key question.

Trauma and Addiction Make It Harder to Stay Safe

Trauma and addiction lead to unsafe behavior even if you don't intend it. You drink more than you planned. You get caught up with people who don't care about you. You don't take care of your body. You isolate. Or you shut down so that you no longer care what happens.

But you can learn to create more safety in your life just as you learned any other subject, such as math or Spanish. You don't have to be an "A" student to do well at it, either. Put your mind to it and keep practicing.

Be kind to yourself as you work on this. You may not have learned to stay safe if you grew up in a family where there was neglect, danger, trauma, or addiction. Your parents couldn't teach you what they didn't know. You may also be mirroring unsafe patterns of friends, community, or culture. Whatever your history, use this chapter to take stock of where you're at now and create an action plan.

✶ Explore . . . *The Safe Behavior Scale*

The scale below is easy to use. You can fill it out weekly to track your score over time.

Be patient with yourself – it may take a while to build greater safety. And for now, *you don't have to decrease any behavior unless you choose to.* The first step is honesty and self-awareness. Later chapters can help you take further action.

The Safe Behavior Scale*

Today's date: _____   Your name or initials: _____

This brief scale helps you build awareness of your safe and unsafe behaviors. If you have trauma or addiction problems, you may feel good but your behavior is unsafe – or the opposite, you may feel bad but your behavior is safe. Behavior "wins" over feelings in providing accurate feedback about your recovery.

Thinking about the past week, in each row circle either "not at all," "some," or "a lot" (don't focus on the numbers for now). Truly *listen* to your behavior – sometimes it may be obvious and other times it may be subtle, perhaps just short of denial.

---

*This scale is reprinted with permission from *Creating Change* by Lisa M. Najavits (forthcoming from The Guilford Press).

Your behavior	Examples	Not at all	Some	A lot	Describe briefly (optional)
1. **Safe coping skills**	Positive use of skills such as asking for help, reading recovery materials, anger management, reducing stress, etc. See "Safe coping skills" (Chapter 12) for more examples.	0	1	2	
2. **Treatment/ self-help groups/ medication**	Actively pursuing structured help (e.g., mental health, substance abuse, medical, dental, self-help groups), attending all as scheduled, and taking all medications as prescribed. ❑ Check here if you have no current need for any of these, and then circle 2 for this item.	0	1	2	
3. **Healthy living**	Good diet, sleep, exercise, balance of work and leisure, etc.	0	1	2	
4. **Major responsibilities**	Fulfilling major duties at work, at school, in your family, etc.	0	1	2	
5. **Daily tasks**	Keeping up with daily to-do's (house cleaning, car upkeep, food shopping, bill paying, staying organized).	0	1	2	
6. **Social support**	Spending time with safe people* (family, friends, colleagues, sponsor, self-help groups); positive and genuine interactions.	0	1	2	
7. **Responding to your feelings**	Staying aware of feelings and responding to them in healthy ways. Includes all types of feelings (e.g., emotions, cravings, body sensations).	0	1	2	
8. **Managing addictive behavior**	Keeping within necessary or agreed-on limits.** For substances, the goal may be abstinence; for spending, it may be a budget, etc.	0	1	2	List the addictive behavior(s) you are rating; and if you circled 0 or 1, describe *how much* and *how often* the behavior(s) occurred***:

Your behavior	Examples	Not at all	Some	A lot	Describe briefly (optional)
9. **Harm to self or others**	Actions such as cutting, burning, suicidal behavior, hitting, punching, yelling, verbal abuse, violence.	2	1	0	If 1 or 0: What type of harm? How much and how often?
10. **Avoiding triggers**	Staying away from trauma and addiction triggers (people, places, and things that are unsafe for you) as much as possible.	0	1	2	
11. **Level of effort**	How much you are actively, strongly, and consistently working to improve your life.	0	1	2	
12. **Other unsafe behavior**	Any other actions that are unsafe for you (e.g., reckless driving, unsafe sex, illegal activity, hanging with unsafe people*).	2	1	0	If 1 or 0: What unsafe behavior(s)? And how much and how often?***

*Unsafe people encourage addictive behavior, put you down, undermine or betray you, physically hurt you, are violent, etc.

**Safe limits on addictive behavior vary by type of addiction and your needs. If you're unclear what's a safe limit for you, get feedback from reputable people or resources.

***List how much the addictive behavior occurred. For example, if you drank, how much did you drink: a bottle of wine? five beers? If you gambled, how much money did you lose? If you watched porn, how many hours did you watch?

How to score it: Add up the numbers you circled (don't be concerned about which column they're listed in). The higher your score, the safer and healthier you are. Track your progress each week to see if you're getting better or worse. Strive to keep increasing your score.

Making it work . . .

- *Be kind to yourself.* See yourself clearly without judgment or blame.

- *Share it with safe, supportive people.* Show your counselor, 12-step sponsor, caring family members, or friends. Also ask them to rate you on the scale and compare your numbers.

- *Make it fun.* Add colors, art, quotes, or anything else that brings it to life.

- *Keep doing it.* Fill it out weekly.

- *Track your scores* on your calendar, phone, or elsewhere to watch your progress.

- *Create a routine.* Try doing it the same time each week and put reminders in place.

- *Stay honest!*

◇ What helps you stay safe?

◇ How can you get yourself to do the Safe Behavior Scale each week?

RECOVERY VOICES

Mike – "I walked into harm's way."

Mike was severely neglected as a child and became addicted to multiple drugs. "As a kid, there was so much danger around me that it seemed normal. When I got older, I worked in construction and would take on terrible jobs that everyone else avoided. I'd walk on icy rooftops. I'd go into dark crawl spaces where there'd be rats. I was so familiar with discomfort that I didn't think twice. The foreman relied on me for that stuff instead of asking the other guys. My counselor helped me see that I was tolerating too much. I began asking the foreman to give the crappy jobs to other guys too. Trauma and addiction had made me so powerless that I didn't protect myself – the gut instinct that flashes 'danger!' was switched off for me. I walked into harm's way, bad situations, and relationships all the time. I was just used to life being hard. This chapter helped me see why I did that. I'm not a stupid person; I'm actually pretty smart. But I hadn't learned how to be safe as a kid. It's like someone who never learned to read and needs to learn it letter by letter as an adult. I'm still learning – I keep taking stock of my decisions to make sure I'm not just going for what feels familiar but going for what's best."

Suggested answers to the quiz in this chapter:

» Safe = items 2, 5, 6, 10, 13, 14, 15, 17, 18, 20, 21

» Unsafe = items 1, 3, 4, 7, 8, 9, 11, 12, 16, 19

8

~∞~

Wish versus reality

Sometimes you have to look reality in the eye and deny it.
—GARRISON KEILLOR, American humorist

Trauma and addiction problems are perpetuated by *not* seeing certain truths. There's a wish to believe things are different than they are. Each person's painful truths are unique, yet there are common themes.

» *Wanting to make it better than it is.* "I'm fine." "He loves me even though he hits me."

» *Wanting control.* "I can quit any time." "I could have saved my buddy if I had been there."

» *Wanting to believe.* "I always told myself I liked my father, but I didn't. I gave him qualities he didn't have, made him different than he was."

» *Wanting it to disappear.* "If I don't think about it, maybe it'll go away."

» *Wanting to be normal.* "It was just part of growing up." "Everyone drinks like this."

» *Wanting it to make sense.* "It's all my fault." "I must have done something to deserve it."

» *Wanting to fit in.* "Everyone else seems fine, so I pretend I am too."

» *Wanting to make it worse than it is.* "Why bother trying? I can't recover."

» *Wanting to be stronger than you are.* "My love will cure him." "I can handle a drink."

» *Any others?* _____

This chapter was adapted with permission from *Creating Change* by Lisa M. Najavits (forthcoming from The Guilford Press).

Courage

It takes real courage to look squarely at trauma and addiction and let yourself see what's really going on. It may feel too hard to admit, "I can never have another drink," or "My mother knew what was going on but didn't stop it." Everything in you may want to fight the truth, may tell you it's too much or too scary, or the flip side, may dismiss it as unimportant. All of these are ways your mind shuts down to protect you from too much truth. You can honor and respect that this helped you survive.

The task now, at your own pace and in your own way, is to let yourself face some of the truths that were too painful to face before. You can decide how, what, and when. This work is often done best in counseling or with the support of people close to you. There's no need to rush or get it all done at once. "Don't take a fence down until you know why it was put up," as the saying goes. And use all the coping skills you can (see "Safe coping skills," Chapter 12).

Know that any truth can be faced. This doesn't mean it's easy; if it were, you'd be doing it already. It may bring up raw feelings like anger and shame. It can make you feel weak or inferior to other people. You may never have learned that facing truth is like pulling off a Band-Aid – it hurts but then gets better. It can lead to good results.

Because your mind tries to protect you from the truth about trauma and addiction, it requires extra effort to shift toward greater awareness. Look for as much factual evidence as you can. Listen to the small, quiet voice within. Hear the feedback of people who know you well.

What It Sounds Like

◇ Look at the following examples – do you see yourself in any of these?

Addiction Examples

Facing the truth	instead of	Not facing the truth
"My liver function test is showing a problem."		"My drinking isn't all that bad."
"I have to start today, even if small steps."		"I'll quit tomorrow."
"I need help."		"I can stop any time I want."

Trauma Examples

Facing the truth	instead of	Not facing the truth
"The flashbacks and nightmares keep happening. I have to work on this."		"If I don't think about it, it'll go away."
"I can't excuse his yelling and hitting me anymore."		"He isn't as bad as people say; I know he loves me."
"Children never deserve abuse no matter what they do."		"If I had been a better child, I wouldn't have been abused."

What It Feels Like

Here's what the process feels like from people who have done it:

» It gets easier the more you do it. Early on, facing a single truth may take huge effort; later, it will come naturally.

» There's a feeling of surrendering to the truth, of letting go.

» It may feel like a weight is lifted. You don't have to keep pretending.

» It's often compared to peeling an onion: each new insight leads to more.

» You may cringe with embarrassment or shame when you see what you've been pushing away.

» It's been called the "point of despair" because at first it may feel awful.

» There are positive feelings, too: clarity in knowing what you need to do next; a sense of pride in facing the truth.

» It is freeing.

Questions That Help

To help overcome the mind's natural tendency to block unpleasant truths, glance through the questions on the next page. You don't have to answer each one – just let yourself gently explore any that feel useful.

» "Can I own my truth even if others disagree?"

» "What messages do I hear – in my behavior, in my body?"

» "Is it taking a toll to keep up a front?"

» "What would my higher power say?"

» "What feedback am I getting from people who truly care about me?"

» "What would it feel like to stop pretending?"

» "The evidence keeps adding up; why do I not want to see it?"

» "Am I hanging on to something that isn't helping me anymore?"

» "What would others say if they saw this?"

» "What would happen if I told myself the truth?"

» "Is there something I'm trying to protect?"

» "What feels too hard to say?"

» "Am I trying to make it better than it really is?"

» "What would it mean if I didn't actually have control?"

» "What feels taboo to think about?"

» "Where am I afraid to go in my own mind?"

✧ How can facing your truths make the future better?

✧ Would it help to work on this chapter with someone else – someone you trust?

✷ Explore . . . *The good that comes from facing your truth*

This exercise focuses on the good that can arise from facing important truths. If you prefer, use the term *owning* or *admitting* instead of *facing*.

Addictive Behavior

1. What's hard for you to face about your **addictive behavior**? _____

_____

2. What **good** can come from facing that truth? _____

_____

EXAMPLE

1. It's hard for me to face that drinking is destroying my marriage. _____

2. The good that can come from this truth is that I can still save my marriage if I take action now, rather than letting things get worse. _____

Trauma

1. What's hard for you to face about your **trauma(s)**? _____

_____

2. What **good** can come from facing that truth? _____

_____

EXAMPLE

1. It's hard for me to face that I wasn't strong enough to fight off my attacker.

2. The good that can come from this truth is that it helps me blame myself less. I was overpowered and did what I could to survive.

RECOVERY VOICES

Samantha − "It grows your compassion."

Samantha endured child abuse, school bullying, and addiction (alcohol, drugs, Internet, and shopping). "It's sad – terribly, horribly sad – how well 'Wish versus Reality' captures what goes on before you can acknowledge the full brunt of reality. Just to keep going you have to pretend sometimes. You can't just sit down on the sidewalk and start screaming. You have to go to work, you have to get on the subway, you have to pay the rent, you have to keep going. Some of the bullying incidents I went through in high school I've kept secret. But recently I've been able to admit what they really were and tell someone else about them. Mostly it's admitting to myself what really happened: being able to say, 'That wasn't teasing. That wasn't joking.' Back then I needed it to be 'teasing'; it couldn't be anything else; absolutely that's what I wanted it to be. That's what I held on to all these years. But that's not what it was at all. It grows your compassion once you admit the reality to yourself and can be gentle with yourself about it. It's kind of surprising, but it turns into a benefit. You work so hard to suppress so much because you think it's too painful to know the truth, but acknowledging the reality is what gives you strength and some positive nourishment of your spirit."

9

Find your way

Each patient carries his own doctor inside.
—Albert Schweitzer, 20th-century German physician and winner
of the Nobel Peace Prize

There are many ways to recover. The phrase *many roads, one journey* captures the idea that there are different paths to the same goal.

In addiction recovery, according to research:

- Some hit bottom; others catch the problem early. ▪ Some use spirituality; others don't. ▪ Some do it a day at a time; others make a commitment for life. ▪ Some use 12-step groups; others don't. ▪ Some get professional help or medication; others don't.

So too in trauma recovery, research shows:

- Some tell their trauma story; others don't. ▪ Some forgive the perpetrator; others never do. ▪ Some get professional help or medication; others don't.

Empowerment

Addiction and trauma are both rooted in powerlessness. Addiction means you can't stop; it has power over you rather than you over it. And no one chooses trauma: whether it's a car accident, assault, natural disaster, sexual violence, or other trauma, the person was powerless to escape.

If your addiction and trauma problems are severe, they undermine your personal power in the world. You may feel like you're lost, just drifting along rather than actively directing your life.

Empowerment is thus hugely important. It means "to give power." It's about having options, choosing what's best for you, saying yes to what helps and no to what doesn't. It's about becoming aware of what you really need and want.

"Everyone Has an Opinion" – Messages You May Hear

Empowerment is especially important when you're confronted with strong or conflicting advice. You may hear many opinions about the "right" way to recover. You may be told you must do things a certain way or seek certain types of help. Even if well intentioned, such perspectives can disempower you. The same advice may have positive impact on one person but negative impact on another. Research shows that there are many ways that work. In the end, it's your life and up to you to decide what works for you.

You may also hear messages that are downright unhelpful even if meant well. Examples relevant to trauma include:

> » "Find something positive in your trauma."
>
> » "Stop thinking about it and it'll go away."
>
> » "Appreciate that it wasn't worse."
>
> » "Time heals all wounds."
>
> » "Everyone has hard times."
>
> » "Just take medication."
>
> » "You have to tell your trauma story to recover."
>
> » "God must be punishing you."
>
> » "You have to confront the perpetrator."
>
> » "You have to forgive the perpetrator."
>
> » "Get clean and sober and then deal with the trauma."
>
> » "Your real problem is addiction, not trauma."

✦ Have you heard any of those messages?

Examples relevant to *addiction* include:

» "If you really wanted to stop, you would."
» "What worked for me will work for you."
» "You have to hit bottom to recover."
» "Taking a psychiatric medication is addiction too."
» "It's simple – just don't pick up the drink."
» "It's all in your genes; you were born that way."
» "If your problem is drugs, it's okay to drink."
» "Gambling isn't a real addiction."
» "Once an addict, always an addict."
» "It's all about your unconscious."
» "You have to go to AA."
» "Your real problem is trauma, not addiction."

✧ Have you heard any of those messages?

What do all of these messages have in common? They're generally not true and not helpful. You may also hear wonderful messages that inspire you. So listen closely and consider your options.

Surprises

How much do you know about getting help for trauma and addiction? Take a look at the points below; there may be some surprises. The term *help* is used here for any type of structured help, including self-help groups and professional care.

✧ Circle any points below that are new to you.

You don't have to admit you have a problem to get help. You may be questioning whether you really have addiction or trauma problems. You don't have to be convinced of it on the front end. The key is to reach out sooner rather than later so that you can figure it out.

Some people get better on their own. Not everyone has to get formal help. Some people are able to do what's called "natural recovery" (they get better on their own). They may be using their existing network of supports such as friends, family, or faith-based communities. They may have strong self-discipline and motivation. But the more severe your problems and the more types of problems you have, the more likely you are to need structured help. If you are trying to get better without formal help, remember to keep observing whether you're getting better or worse (see "Listen to your behavior," Chapter 7).

Old-style harsh confrontation of addiction is not recommended. The classic image of in-your-face addiction treatment ("Tear 'em down to build 'em up") is no longer recommended. Now the idea is compassionate support plus accountability. You still have to do what it takes to get better, but the approach shouldn't involve belittling or berating you.

Telling your trauma story isn't enough. Many people believe that if they can just purge or spill their story they'll feel better. But it's not a toxin you expel and then it's gone. It's more than just the facts of what happened; it's also about the meanings it holds for you, feelings that come up, and how it relates to other problems, including addiction. See "Two types of trauma counseling" (Chapter 33) for more.

You don't have to feel motivated for treatment to work. You just have to show up. Motivation sometimes happens along the way rather than at the start. If you feel hope-less or depressed, it can take a while to get energized toward recovery goals. Good care, whether professional or self-help, starts where you're at and helps inspire your motivation.

Start early; don't wait until you "hit bottom." Like physical problems such as cancer or diabetes, early care is best. Hitting bottom can lead to change but is not required. The sooner you start, the better (see "How do people change?" Chapter 5). For addiction, resources such as Rethinking Drinking and Moderation Management are designed to provide help early on (see "Resources," Appendix B).

There's no addictive personality. It's now understood, based on decades of research, that people with addiction have many types of personalities. Addiction isn't a personality problem; it's a medical illness that arises from genes and life experiences (including your peer group, stress, trauma, culture, etc.).

How you feel by the third session of counseling predicts how you'll feel about it months and even years later. Do you feel a positive bond with the counselor and the treatment? If it's not there by the third session, discuss it with the counselor and/or shop around (see "Find a good counselor," Chapter 32).

You can combine any mix of help that you choose. There's often benefit, and no known harm, from getting different types of help at the same time, such as counseling, self-help groups, and medication. In general, the more the better.

If you're forced into addiction treatment, you're just as likely to succeed as those who attend on their own. It's often believed that people have to want help or it won't work. But research shows that people who are forced to attend, such as by the courts or an employer, do just as well as those who choose to attend. However, the same is not true for trauma treatment – in general, it's not recommended to force a person into that.

Twelve-step groups can be great, but other approaches also work. Twelve-step groups help millions of people and are an extraordinary free resource. But there are also other paths for successful recovery, including nonspiritual methods such as SMART Recovery.

You may be able to reduce addictive behavior rather than fully give it up – but be careful. This has been studied most in relation to alcohol and gambling. If you have early or less serious problems, you may be able to return to safe levels, called *controlled use.* But if you have a serious or long-standing addiction, you usually need to stop altogether, called *abstinence.* This is a tricky issue, so get advice from good sources. Abstinence is always safer, so if in doubt go with that. And of course, for some addictions, such as food or work, abstinence is not possible.

You don't have to do it for yourself. It's terrific if you want to help yourself. But if not, you can use whatever you care most about to steer yourself toward recovery. Some people do it for their kids or a partner. That can work for now, and eventually you may find the motivation deep within you.

You don't have to be "clean and sober" before working on trauma. If you have both addiction and trauma problems, working on them at the same time can boost your recovery. The key is *how* you work on them. There are two basic ways to address trauma: focusing on the present or on the past (or sometimes a mix of these). See "Two types of trauma counseling" (Chapter 33) to explore what may be best for you.

Most formal help performs equally well – so choose what you like. "Formal help" here refers to specific models that have been scientifically tested. You may be surprised to hear that although there are different brand names they all perform about equally well. This is called *distinctions without a difference* – although the names of the approaches differ, their power to help you is basically the same. Yet they may differ in other important ways such as cost (some are more expensive); appeal (you may prefer one approach to another); and access (some can be done by peers; others require professionals). For example, 12-step models do as well as professional therapies in their results.

You can attend 12-step groups even if you don't believe you have an addiction. They're free, and anyone can go to open meetings. You'll hear people talk about their "experience, strength, and hope." You don't have to speak. You can go before you have a major addiction problem to prevent it from getting worse.

Consider medications. There are various medications for trauma and/or addiction problems, including some that help your mood and some that decrease cravings.

If you have both trauma and addiction problems, you may need different help. Some medications for trauma, such as benzodiazepines, may not be a good choice, as they can become addictive. Trauma counseling that focuses on the past (telling the trauma story) may be too intense if you have current severe addiction (see "Two types of trauma counseling," Chapter 33). But in general, people with both trauma and addiction problems benefit from many different types of help, including 12-step groups.

The more help you get and the longer you attend, the better the results. But find the best help you can. Keep noticing how it makes you feel. Good help can be so very healing, but poor-quality help may be worse than no help. Don't stay in treatment that is harmful to you.

Help Comes in Many Packages

"The main message was that they cared about me and that, no matter what, they would help me. . . . They seemed to like me even though I didn't like myself. They kind of loved me back to life again."
  —From *The Breaking the Cycle Compendium: Vol. 1. The Roots of Relationship* by Margaret Leslie

---

There are many formats and types of help. To the extent that you can, choose what appeals to you. And remember – in general, the more help the better.

✧ As you go through the next four sections, mark any types of help that you're willing to try.

Different Formats

» *Self-help groups* are free and consist of peers helping each other.

» *Guided self-change* allows you to set goals for yourself and pursue them on your own.

» *Professional counseling* can be individual and/or group.

» *Medication.*

» *Self-help books.*

» *Online groups and supports.*

» *Treatment programs* such as rehab, a day program, or hospital.

» *Community supports* such as a sober house or job program.

» *Body-focused work* such as yoga and acupuncture.

Different Approaches to Trauma

» *Present-focused counseling*: emphasis on the present; learning new skills and information to cope with current trauma problems.

» *Past-focused counseling*: emphasis on the past, such as telling the story of your trauma in detail and exploring your feelings about it.

» *A combination of present- and past-focused counseling:* See "Two types of trauma counseling" (Chapter 33) for more on present- versus past-focused trauma counseling and names of specific models.

» *Trauma-informed care*: a treatment program in which all staff are trained to understand trauma. The goal is compassionate care (no harsh confrontation or coercion) and strong attention to trauma (evaluating all clients for trauma and providing trauma services).

Different Approaches to Addiction

» *Abstinence*: the goal is to give up the addictive behavior completely – for addictions where this is possible, such as substances and gambling.

» *Harm reduction*: gradually decreasing the addictive behavior with the idea that "50% of something is better than 100% of nothing."

» *Controlled use*: the idea is that some people, such as those with mild addiction, can return to safe levels of use.

See "Tip the Scales recovery plan" (Chapter 21) for more on those three approaches.

» *Spiritually based programs* such as 12-step groups that emphasize a higher power or church-based models such as Celebrate Recovery.

» *Changing thinking and behavior,* such as SMART Recovery, Rethinking Drinking, and Moderation Management, relapse prevention, and cognitive-behavioral therapy.

» *Physical testing* (urine, breath, hair, blood) can be used to monitor substance use. Urine testing is the most common and has become so inexpensive that it can be done at home, such as for a parent who wants to monitor a teenager.

» *Addiction-informed care* is not a widely used term but can be used to identify treatment programs that provide best-practice approaches to addiction. All staff are trained in addiction and provide a compassionate approach to it; all clients are evaluated for addiction and quality addiction services are provided.

Different Approaches for Trauma plus Addiction

If you have both addiction and trauma problems, there are yet more options:

» *Integrated care* addresses trauma and addiction at the same time, by the same counselor. The most widely used and studied is Seeking Safety (*www.seekingsafety.org*). See "Two types of trauma counseling" (Chapter 33) for other models.

» *Sequential care* focuses first on one and then on the other (typically addiction first, then trauma).

» *Parallel care* provides help for both at the same time but by two different counselors or programs. You might be in an addiction program and receive trauma counseling from an outside counselor, for example.

Who, Not Just *What* –
The Helper Is as Important as the Model

If you do seek help, whether from professionals or self-help groups, the "who" matters too. You may go to one AA group and get a lot from it and go to another and get little. Try different groups until you find ones that suit you. Shop around for professional help too, such as counseling. Some people spend a lot of time with nice, kind counselors who aren't effective, so make sure you feel a good connection *and* that you're making real progress with measurable changes (see "Find a good counselor," Chapter 32).

Evidence-Based Care

Evidence-based care refers to formal help that has been scientifically studied. Yet such studies look at averages: how well treatments work across a large number of people. Individuals vary amid those averages. What works for you may not work for someone else. Also the field is young; new studies are being done all the time, and the quality of studies is improving. Some studies in the past were small or did not include important subgroups, such as women, adolescents, or diverse ethnicities. To explore the evidence for various types of help, see "Resources," Appendix B. You can learn how to search for free, accurate medical information about treatment. If you are currently in counseling, you can ask your counselor about the evidence for the approach being used. But there are also excellent types of help that have not yet been formally studied, so stay aware of how helpful it feels (see "Find a good counselor," Chapter 32).

✱ Explore . . . *12 questions to ask when seeking help*

The more you understand on the front end, the better. Some questions you can ask when exploring formal help:

1. If I were to relapse in my addiction, what would happen? (Some programs may ask you to leave while others will let you stay.)

2. How long will it take?

3. How much does it cost? Do you accept my insurance?

4. How will I know if I'm getting better?

5. Does your approach have a name? Can I read more about it online?

6. Will I be required to share my trauma story in detail? What if I prefer not to?

7. What is your perspective on working on trauma and addiction at the same time?

8. Is there any research on your type of help? (There may not be research, but if it exists it's good to know about.)

9. How will you identify what types of problems I have?

10. Will I have a choice of who I work with? Can I switch if it doesn't feel like a good fit?

11. If I don't improve or worsen, what are my options?

12. Are there any requirements, such as attending AA or anything else?

Finding Your Way

The title of this chapter has layers of meaning. It's about finding *your* way – what you uniquely need. It's about finding your *way* – as in a maze, you may go down some blind alleys but can keep searching for a good path. So "figure out who you are and do it on purpose." Life becomes more manageable and joyful when you accept the reality of yourself and the world and integrate them in positive ways.

RECOVERY VOICES

David – "There just might be a way out."

"I love this chapter for the simple reason that trauma and addiction are indeed absolute powerlessness, and information and options give me a little hope that there just might be a way out. There's so much misinformation about how to get well. Having experienced numerous psych hospitals, detoxes, halfway houses, rehabs, a therapeutic community, and a lot of therapy – some of it good, some of it bad – not to mention being prescribed a host of psych meds, I can safely say that what works for one person doesn't necessarily work for another. This chapter is full of great suggestions. The ideas on how to choose a therapist and what questions to ask when seeking help take some of the guesswork out of the process. I also like that a lot of different paths are listed because that makes me feel like I do have choices and some control. My experience with trauma and addiction is that they sap all motivation to make changes, so it was helpful to read that action often precedes motivation. I think I'd use "Listen to your behavior" (Chapter 7) to identify my most severe negative behaviors and then use this chapter to get in touch with what I want to do for next steps. I take an active role in designing my recovery program."

10

Possible selves

Most of us have two lives – the life we live and the unlived life
within us.
—STEVEN PRESSFIELD, American author

We all have various possible selves, both ones we hope to become and ones we dread
becoming. "The possible selves that are hoped for might include the successful self,
the creative self, the rich self, the thin self, or the loved and admired self, whereas the
dreaded possible selves could be the alone self, the depressed self, the incompetent
self, the alcoholic self, the unemployed self, or the bag lady self," said Hazel Markus
and Paula Nurius in an article in *American Psychologist*.

Situations can bring out better and worse versions of you. This is hopeful because
it means that even if you feel bad about yourself now, that can change. You can gain
or regain the best sides of yourself. Sustained recovery means the best sides of you are
"driving the car" enough to stay on the right road.

With trauma and addiction you may be cut off from yourself, unsure what you
feel, unsure what matters. You may watch yourself doing things you don't want to be
doing or just not caring anymore. As you work on recovery you'll find greater wholeness: the ability to sustain a better version of yourself and one larger than trauma and
addiction.

Best Self (in Recovery)

I hope to become someone who . . .

    . . . can have impulses without acting on them.
    . . . finds trustworthy people to be with.
    . . . is responsible.

. . . is a loving parent.

. . . takes good care of myself.

. . . says what I need and want.

. . . has healthy closeness with others.

. . . _____ [fill in your own].

✧ Which *best self* statements matter to you?

Worst Self (Not in Recovery)

I dread being someone who . . .

. . . lies to people who love me.

. . . lashes out at others.

. . . gets into dangerous situations.

. . . doesn't care anymore.

. . . lets my addiction take over.

. . . can't set boundaries.

. . . becomes numb.

. . . _____ [fill in your own].

✧ Which *worst self* statements matter to you?

Research shows that people who (1) imagine a better possible self *and* (2) identify specific ways to move toward it are the most likely to achieve that better self. Both parts are needed.

For example, a study by Daphna Oyserman and colleagues focused on 160 school-age low-income disadvantaged youth. They used a simple exercise like the one that follows. Those who (1) imagined a best possible academic self in the next school year *and* (2) had specific strategies to achieve it did better in school months later than those who had only "1," the positive vision alone.

Also, it can help to think of various categories of possible selves to explore:

» An *emotional* possible self (how you respond to your feelings).

» A *relationship* possible self (how you respond to others).

» A *work or school* self (your achievement goals).

» A *spiritual* possible self (how you relate to a higher connection).

» A *physical* possible self (diet, exercise, etc.).

» A *recovery* possible self (trauma/addiction).

Examples of "Who I hope to become"

- "I hope to become a graduate student in a social work program," "I hope to become abstinent from cocaine," "I hope to lose 20 pounds," "I hope to become leader of my division at work," "I hope to become a partner in a loving relationship," "I hope to become someone who meditates daily," "I hope to be someone who keeps promises," "I hope to become a parent."

Examples of "Who I dread becoming"

- "I dread getting divorced," "I dread becoming homeless," "I dread becoming a chronic alcoholic," "I dread losing my job," "I dread going to jail," "I dread becoming a college dropout," "I dread being a bad parent."

⋆ Explore . . . *Your possible selves*

This exercise is adapted from Oyserman and colleagues' Possible Selves Questionnaire. First is an example and then a blank version for you to fill out.

Example: *Best Self*

Question 1: *Who do you hope to become?*

(a) Picture yourself a year from now. Who do you hope to become?

- *By next year I hope to become someone who <u>keeps control of my temper.</u>*

(b) What are you doing now to become that person, if anything? (List whatever is true.)

- *<u>I'm taking a class in anger management.</u>*
- *<u>I'm asking my doctor to change my medications.</u>*

(c) What more could you do to become that person? (List as many options as you can.)

- *I could read a self-help book about it.*
- *I could pray on it.*
- *I could try practicing relaxation when I get angry.*

Your Turn: *Best Self*

Question 1: *Who do you hope to become?*

(a) Picture yourself a year from now. Who do you hope to become?

- *By next year I would like to become someone who* _____.

(b) What are you doing now to become that person, if anything? (List whatever is true.)

- _____
- _____
- _____

(c) What more could you be doing to become that person? (List as many options as you can.)

- _____
- _____
- _____
- _____

Example: *Worst Self*

Question 2: *Who do you dread becoming?*

(a) Picture yourself a year from now. Who do you dread becoming?

- *By next year I dread becoming <u>unable to pay my bills.</u>*

(b) What are you doing now to avoid becoming that person, if anything? (List whatever is true.)

- *<u>I'm not doing anything about it even though I know I should be.</u>*

(c) What more could you be doing now to avoid becoming that person? (List as many options as you can.)

- *<u>I could prepare a budget.</u>*
- *<u>I could set aside money in savings.</u>*

- *I could read books on how to manage finances.*
- *I could stop buying clothes I don't need.*

Your Turn: *Worst Self*

Question 2: *Who do you dread becoming?*

    (a) Picture yourself a year from now. Who do you dread becoming?

- *By next year I dread becoming someone who* _____.

    (b) What are you doing now to avoid becoming that person, if anything? (List whatever is true.)

- _____
- _____
- _____

    (c) What more could you be doing now to avoid becoming that person? (List as many options as you can.)

- _____
- _____
- _____
- _____

✧ What will you do today to move *toward* your best self?

✧ What will you do today to move *away from* your worst self?

RECOVERY VOICES

David – "I mold myself into the man I want to become."

"This chapter is short but so important. I'll use the exercise to envision who I want to become but tie that into being compassionate and accepting of myself for being where I am now. I think the hardest thing for me to do when I'm using drugs or not feeling and acting the way I want to is to say to myself, 'Dave, I love you and accept you right now; right in this moment I love you and accept you.'

I vacillate between so many emotions that it's hard sometimes to really have a sense of myself. And if I don't know who I am, how can I possibly love myself? I like that this chapter helps me move past the false belief that I am my trauma or I am my addiction. I can look at the exercise and pick something from it to practice. If I want to be the kind of person who takes a walk every day, then I need to go for a walk. Each day I might take one item from the exercise and work on it. Thinking about my best and worst possible selves feels empowering – I take control of my transformation, molding myself into the man I want to become."

11

The language of trauma and addiction

The limits of my language are the limits of my world.
—LUDWIG WITTGENSTEIN, 20th-century Austrian philosopher

Do you speak the language of trauma and addiction recovery?

Language is far more than a tool – it shapes how you think and feel, how you relate to people, and how you interpret your experiences. It reflects culture of all kinds, including those of your family and community. Trauma and addiction are often misunderstood, which gets reflected in language too.

⟡ Notice how you feel when you read row 1 versus row 2.

Row 1: *junkie; boozer; crazy; freak; low-life; drama-queen; unstable; misfit*

Row 2: *drug problem; trauma survivor; mentally ill; disadvantaged; PTSD; bullied*

Jennyfer, who survived a stray bullet, says, "I've removed the word *victim* from my vocabulary when describing myself and replaced it with *survivor*. That one small tweak changes my whole story from a tragedy to a triumph and helps me reclaim my power."

This chapter offers a list of key terms relevant to addiction and trauma recovery. They are more than just jargon – they reflect important ideas that can help you better understand yourself. Accurate language also helps you build a healthy perspective:

you're not the problem; rather, you have problems based on your experiences. The more you learn, the stronger you become.

By searching for the answers rather than reading a list of definitions, you'll get a deeper sense of what they mean and how they relate to your recovery. The best way to search is online, entering each term, seeing where it leads you, and following the trail further if it sparks your interest. Beyond formal definitions, you can also explore other people's perspectives and locate resources for help. If you're not familiar with how to search online, go to a public library and have a librarian show you. It's easy and will open up new worlds for you.

You can also play the lists as a scavenger hunt with other people; see the game rules at the end of the chapter.

Try to explore the concepts in a felt, emotional way, rather than a dry, technical way. The best thinking involves both the head and the heart. Notice what moves you, what piques your interest. This isn't school – it's life.

✫ Explore . . . *Addiction language*

1. Tolerance

2. Withdrawal

3. "Pink cloud"

4. Medication-assisted treatment

5. The 12 steps (list all of them)

6. Chasing losses

7. Abstinence violation effect

8. Natural recovery

9. Urge-surfing

10. Symptom substitution

11. Controlled use

12. Harm reduction

13. Abstinence

14. "Dry but not sober"

15. Denial

16. Enabling

17. Al-Anon

18. SMART Recovery

19. Slip versus relapse

20. Hitting bottom

21. Polysubstance use

22. Self-medication

23. Others? _____

✴ Explore . . . *Trauma language*

1. Dissociation

2. Trauma-informed care

3. Splitting

4. Re-experiencing

5. Intergenerational trauma

6. Flashback

7. Retraumatization

8. Betrayal trauma

9. Moral injury

10. Acute stress disorder

11. Anniversary reaction

12. Boundaries

13. Grounding

14. Trauma

15. Posttraumatic stress disorder (PTSD)

16. Foreshortened future

17. Hypervigilance

18. Avoidance

19. Secondary trauma

20. Complex trauma

21. Reenactment

22. Simple trauma

23. Others? _____

✸ Explore ... *The Scavenger Hunt Game*

This game uses the terms from *addiction language* and *trauma language* above. It is called a scavenger hunt because it's played like one except instead of searching for physical objects the search is for definitions. The game can be played by two or more people.

1. The game leader decides on a time period, which can be any length that makes sense for you (an hour, day, week, etc.).

2. Split into two or more teams. *Note*: If there are just two people, each person is a team. A maximum of five people per team is suggested. Teams can give themselves a name if they choose to.

3. Each team huddles and decides how to get working on finding as many right answers as possible for each list above (addiction language, trauma language). Team members can draw on their own knowledge and/or search online or at a library. Each team can do the items in the list in any order (they don't have to start with 1 and go through 22). Also for question 23 the team gets a point for any additional term they list and define.

4. When the time is up, the two teams come together to score their answers. The team with the most right answers wins the game. How can you know if an answer is right? Read each answer out loud, and if anyone challenges the answer, believing it to be inaccurate, the game leader checks the answer online.

Variation: Real versus fake answers. A twist on the game is to allow the teams to offer fake answers that sound real, which is like the game Dictionary (also known as Balderdash or Fictionary). You can look up the rules for those online and apply them to the addiction/trauma terms in this chapter.

Good luck and good learning.

RECOVERY VOICES

Sabrina − "This is how we do it; this is how we get better."

Sabrina survived child abuse and neglect and struggled with substance and shopping addiction as well as food issues. "Some of these terms I didn't know, so I looked them up, like *abstinence violation effect* and *urge-surfing*. Urge-surfing is really good for me, as I recently stopped taking diet pills. All day yesterday for me was about getting through whatever I was feeling, which was mostly anger at not being able to do what I wanted. I get this roaring type of anger − not at anyone, not lashing out but a kind of ferocious roar − and I found the urge-surfing helped me get through it so I could keep moving forward. What I like about this chapter is that it's knowledge that I can use right away. Just knowing more about what's going on gives me more control over my behavior. I also like how it doesn't give the definitions but lets me figure how the concepts apply to me instead of authorities telling me a single notion of what they mean. This is how we do it, this is how we get better – we incorporate what we're being taught and make it our own. Some of the concepts are very rich and I want to read more about them, like *moral injury*. I think the scavenger hunt game might be fun to try too."

12

Safe coping skills

> We all have problems. The way we solve them is what makes us different.
> —UNKNOWN

Coping means how you respond to problems – how you try to solve them.

Picture yourself going through a painful divorce. Poor coping would be drinking a lot, isolating, and gaining weight on junk food. These short-term fixes worsen problems. Good coping might be joining a support group and taking care of yourself by getting sleep and exercise. These help in the long term.

In short, *you can't always control what happens, but you can choose how you respond.* Strive for solutions that build strength and healing. As long as it's safe – not hurting yourself or anyone else – it's good coping.

Trauma and addiction make it difficult to cope well. But good coping can be learned. This chapter offers a list of more than 80 safe coping skills relevant to trauma and addiction. The list was published in the book *Seeking Safety* (*www.seekingsafety. org*) and has been used all over the world. Add your own safe coping skills to the list – there are as many ways of coping safely as there are people. Find what works for you and let go of the rest. Many people find it helpful to carry around a copy of the list as a reminder.

✶ Explore . . . *The Safe Coping Skills List*

Put a star next to new coping skills you want to try; put a checkmark next to those you're already good at. Experiment with all sorts of skills. Remember, too, that context matters: a skill that is healthy in one setting may not be in another. If you don't understand some of the skills, ask a counselor or trusted person to help you.

Safe Coping Skills

1. Ask for help: Reach out to someone safe.   **2. Inspire yourself:** Carry something positive (e.g., poem) or negative (e.g., photo of friend who overdosed).   **3. Leave a bad scene:** When things go wrong, get out.   **4. Persist:** Never, never, never, never, never, never, never, never give up.   **5. Honesty:** Secrets and lying are at the core of trauma and addiction; honesty heals them.   **6. Cry:** Let yourself cry; it will not last forever.   **7. Choose self-respect:** Choose whatever will make you like yourself tomorrow.   **8. Take good care of your body:** Healthy eating, exercise, safe sex.   **9. List your options:** In any situation, you have choices.   **10. Create meaning:** Remind yourself what you are living for: your children? love? truth? justice? God?   **11. Do the best you can with what you have:** Make the most of available opportunities.   **12. Set a boundary:** Say "no" to protect yourself.   **13. Compassion:** Listen to yourself with respect and care.   **14. When in doubt, do what's hardest:** The most difficult path is invariably the right one.   **15. Talk yourself through it:** Self-talk helps in difficult times.   **16. Imagine:** Create a mental picture that helps you to feel different (e.g., remember a safe place).   **17. Notice the choice point:** In slow motion, notice the exact moment when you chose unsafe behavior.   **18. Pace yourself:** If overwhelmed, go slower; if stagnant, go faster.   **19. Stay safe:** Do whatever you need to do to put your safety above all.   **20. Seek understanding, not blame:** Listen to your behavior; blaming prevents growth.   **21. If one way doesn't work, try another:** As if in a maze, turn a corner and try a new path.   **22. Link trauma and addiction:** Recognize addiction as an attempt to soothe emotional pain.   **23. Alone is better than a bad relationship:** If only treaters are safe for now, that's okay.   **24. Create a new story:** You are the author of your life: be the hero who overcomes adversity.   **25. Avoid avoidable suffering:** Prevent bad situations in advance.   **26. Ask others:** Ask others if your belief is accurate.   **27. Get organized:** You'll feel more in control with "to-do" lists and a clean house.   **28. Watch for danger signs:** Face a problem before it becomes huge; notice red flags.   **29. Healing above all:** Focus on what matters.   **30. Try something, anything:** A good plan today is better than a perfect one tomorrow.   **31. Discovery:** Find out whether your assumption is true rather than staying "in your head."   **32. Attend treatment:** AA, self-help, counseling, medications, groups – anything that keeps you going.   **33. Create a buffer:** Put something between you and danger (e.g., time, distance).   **34. Say what you really think:** You'll feel closer to others (but only do this with safe people).   **35. Listen to your needs:** No more neglect – really hear what you need.   **36. Move toward your opposite:** For example, if you are too dependent try being more independent.   **37. Replay the scene:** Review a negative event: What can you do differently next time?   **38. Notice the cost:** What is the price of addiction in your life?   **39. Structure your day:** A productive schedule keeps you on track and connected to the world.   **40. Set an action plan:** Be specific, set a deadline, and let others know about it.   **41. Protect yourself:** Put up a shield against destructive people, bad environments, and addiction.   **42. Soothing talk:** Talk to yourself very gently (as if to a friend or small child).   **43. Think of the consequences:** Really see the impact for tomorrow, next week, next year.   **44. Trust the process:** Just keep moving forward; the only way out is through.   **45. Work the material:** The more you practice and participate, the quicker the healing.   **46. Integrate the split self:** Accept all sides of yourself; they are there for a reason.   **47. Expect growth to feel uncomfortable:** If it feels awkward or difficult, you're doing it right.   **48. Replace destructive activities:** Eat candy instead of getting high.   **49. Pretend you like yourself:** See how different the day feels.   **50. Focus on now:** Do what you can to make today better; don't get overwhelmed by the past or future.   **51. Praise yourself:** Notice what you did right; this is the most powerful method of growth.   **52. Observe repeating patterns:** Try to notice and understand your reenactments.   **53. Self-nurture:** Do something that you enjoy (e.g., take a walk, see a movie).   **54. Practice delay:** If you can't totally prevent a self-destructive act, at least delay it as long as possible.   **55. Let go of destructive relationships:** If it can't be fixed, detach.   **56. Take responsibility:** Take an active, not a passive approach.   **57. Set a deadline:** Make it happen by setting a date.   **58. Make a commitment:** Promise yourself to do what's right to help your recovery.   **59. Rethink:** Think in a way that helps you feel better.   **60. Detach from emotional pain (grounding):** Distract, walk away, change the channel.   **61. Learn from experience:** Seek wisdom that can help you next time.   **62. Solve the problem:** Don't take it personally when things go wrong – try just to seek a solution.   **63. Use kinder language:** Make your language less harsh.   **64. Examine the evidence:** Evaluate both sides of the issue.   **65. Plan it out:** Take the time to think ahead – it's the opposite of impulsivity.   **66. Identify the belief:** Examples: shoulds, deprivation reasoning.   **67. Reward yourself:** Find a healthy way to celebrate anything you do right.   **68. Create a new script:** Rehearse new ways of thinking.   **69. Find rules to live by:** Remember a phrase that works for you (e.g., "Stay real").   **70. Setbacks are not failures:** A setback is just a setback, nothing more.   **71. Tolerate the feeling:** "No feeling is final" – just get through it safely.   **72. Actions first, and feelings will follow:** Don't wait until you feel motivated; just start now.   **73. Create positive addictions:** Examples: sports, hobbies, AA. . . .   **74. When in doubt, don't:** If you suspect danger, stay away.   **75. Fight the trigger:** Take an active approach to protect yourself.   **76. Notice the source:** Before you accept criticism or advice, notice who's telling it to you.   **77. Make a decision:** If you're stuck, try choosing the best solution you can right now; don't wait.   **78. Do the right thing:** Do what you know will help you even if you don't feel like it.   **79. Go to a meeting:** Feet first; just get there and let the rest happen.   **80. Protect your body from HIV:** This is truly an important issue.   **81. Prioritize healing:** Make healing your most urgent and important goal, above all else.   **82. Reach for community resources:** Lean on them! They can be a source of great support.   **83. Get others to support your recovery:** Tell people what you need.   **84. Notice what you can control:** List the aspects of your life you do control (e.g., job, friends . . .).

Keep It Visible

- In your wallet (good coping is worth more than money).
- On your mirror (reflect who you're becoming).
- On your refrigerator (serve up healthy coping).
- Or anywhere else that keeps it visible – your phone, car, or elsewhere.

✧ What safe coping skills can you use today?

✧ Where can you keep this list so you'll remember to keep using it?

✧ Do you notice any positive feelings as you go through the list?

✧ Are there other safe coping skills you use that aren't on this list?

RECOVERY VOICES

Brianna – "I have a choice here."

"Here's what the coping skills are for me: I get triggered, I take a breath, and I say, 'I have a choice here.' I survived terrible trauma as a kid and reacted to it by buying stuff to fill the emptiness inside. I was addicted to external things. I always had a beautiful sports car, clothes, all of that stuff. I had huge amounts of *things*. But I finally really got what people say – nothing on the outside is gonna fill you up. Stuff doesn't work. You can try it over and over until you create financial destruction. That's what happened to me – my devastating financial situation caused a whole lot of pain and I finally saw that my way of coping was unsafe. When I saw the list of safe coping skills, I thought, 'This is it.' Healing really happens when you understand that you can *choose* how you respond to what happens in the world. When I fully owned that, it was huge. I love the list of safe coping skills because it's practical. I wanted ideas for what to do, especially when things were unsafe and I was being bombarded and couldn't understand the cause and effect – why things kept falling apart. I kept thinking it was because of other people until I realized it was me that had to start doing something different. I got that loud and clear. Because of my financial problems I had lost my car, so I had to take the bus. I took the list of safe coping skills in my backpack. Every day for about 6 months I'd pull it out on the bus and work on a few skills. I'd say, 'How do I use this one?' I found it important to do lots of examples. I'd also pick out my top skills and make flashcards with them and make them attractive with some art so I'd want to use them; I kept those in my backpack too. The safe coping skills are the essence of recovery because you can sit forever and think about recovery, but it's like AA says: feet first. Get your body there and your mind will follow. You've got to *do* the coping. When you start to do it, you start to have positive results, and when you have positive results you want to do it more."

13

Social pain

> The biggest disease today is not leprosy or tuberculosis, but rather the feeling of being unwanted.
>
> −MOTHER TERESA, 20th-century Albanian missionary and winner of the Nobel Peace Prize

When most people think of pain, they picture physical pain, such as a broken bone or a migraine. But pain can be not only physical but emotional, spiritual, and social too.

Social pain is what you feel when you or others are subjected to injustice, betrayal, discrimination, isolation, persecution, racism, exclusion, or other forms of social suffering. In some situations, such as gang life, wartime, or sick family environments, you may have been forced to cause harm to others, which can also result in intense social pain.

Trauma and addiction are often bound up in social pain too. You may be unfairly blamed for your trauma or addiction. You may be demeaned or rejected for having problems. Your trauma or addiction may occur in relationships where you're mistreated. The list goes on and on.

Tanya: "As I grew up I knew I wasn't a boy, even if I didn't have the words until I was older. My father tried to beat me into being a boy. His message was 'You're no good.' I carried that message into a life of shame – homelessness, prostitution, crack addiction. But I had an aunt who loved me for who I was. After leaving home and discovering who I am – a woman (I made the outward change in my 30s) – she's been right there with me, a buffer to what I hear and have heard from my family, my community, the world. It's taken a while, but I've been able to shed the old messages and old ways of living. I'm sober. I no longer seek money from my sugar daddy. I'm in a loving relationship, full of zest for life!"

✧ Do you feel rejected, put down, bullied, humiliated, or shunned as part of
   trauma, addiction, or other experiences?

✧ Do you feel isolated, unique, or misunderstood because of what you lived
   through?

✧ Have you had to watch other people being seriously harmed or mistreated?

✧ Do you feel lonely a lot?

✧ Are you haunted by having done things that hurt other people?

✧ Does the term *social pain* make sense to you even without fully reading this
   chapter?

Social Pain Is Real

Social pain is as real as physical pain, according to studies of brain imaging. It occurs
at all level of society: in families, peer groups, and institutions such as the church,
military, corporations, and schools. It occurs via social media too, such as online bullying, which causes as much harm as direct social contact, according to research.

Social pain can have serious consequences:

» It can make you physically ill by weakening your immune system.

» It triggers aggression; you may fight to gain respect or lash out at someone who
  hurt you.

» It can distort self-perception: "I walk down the street, and people can tell I was
  abused as a kid."

» It leads to isolation.

Margaret joined the Army after 9/11. Her father had served in Navy peacekeeping
missions, and her grandfather fought in World War II. She got outstanding reviews
by her superiors and was respected by peers. She wanted a lifelong military career

but left after 5 years. "By then, I wasn't the same person who had joined. My career went into a nosedive after I reported being raped by my commanding officer. People who used to respect me snubbed me. It's like they thought I made it up. There were rumors and some really disgusting jokes. Everyone seemed to know about the rape, even though it was supposed to be confidential. I got assigned to a new unit, and the commander there was told that I was now 'their problem.' There was never a real investigation into what happened, so I finally left. I was shocked that I could be so quickly tossed aside after all that training and all my successes. I was seen as 'this bitch who lied.' The hero became the nobody."

Many Pathways

Social pain occurs in numerous ways.

- » *Not being believed.* You may have been told, "You're making it up," or "It wasn't so bad." Such invalidation is all the more painful if it comes from parents or other authority figures who are supposed to be there for you.

- » *Humiliation.* Being made fun of, publicly shamed, debased, degraded, or told you're less than other people can cause lasting impact.

- » *Betrayal.* You may have trusted someone who turned on you. It can be devastating to have your secrets shared with others or to be lied to about important matters.

- » *Isolation.* If you were isolated during or after trauma or addiction, you may never have received support for recovery. You may feel misunderstood or doubt your own reality.

- » *Taboos.* Traumas like incest, torture, and genocide are so extreme that others may turn away or deny them. Addictions that are socially unacceptable can also evoke rejection.

- » *Scapegoating.* You may have been singled out for harm while others weren't. One child in a family may be abused while the others aren't. In the Holocaust, Jews and gays were targeted, for example. Scapegoating is always unfair.

- » *Forced to harm others.* You may feel deep social pain if you had to hurt others and didn't want to, such as atrocities during war or being forced to hurt a sibling as part of child abuse.

- » *Blame.* You may be blamed for what happened even if you had no control over it. In some cultures rape victims are shunned by their family and community. These distortions of truth are deeply destructive.

✧ Are any descriptions above familiar to you?

What to Do about It

There are no simple solutions, but here are some ideas.

People cause social pain, but they can heal it too. The more you find good decent people who respect you, the more you can overcome social pain. It can be hard to find such people, but even one trusted person can make a difference – a friend, counselor, family, teacher, or religious figure. Who can you reach out to even if it means starting with a total stranger, such as a hotline or crisis center?

You can use nonsocial methods too. Anything that builds your life in a positive direction will help; you don't have to solve social pain through social means. Nature, art, learning, physical activity, and other endeavors can offer new dimensions that shrink down the importance of social pain.

If possible, find new social environments where you may be treated differently. This may mean changing schools, leaving a job, or moving. But leaving isn't always a solution – if you keep changing environments and the same patterns arise, learn new skills to protect yourself more (see "Perception: How others view you," Chapter 27).

Know that it's not just you. Social pain leads to isolation; you may feel like you're the only one who's humiliated and rejected. But sadly, the history of the world is full of social pain. Strive to understand all you can about it – why it's so common and how it plays out in different contexts. Seeing it with open eyes strengthens you.

Keep your idealism, but be realistic. Social pain can destroy your ideals about fairness, justice, and goodness in others. You may feel blindsided by meanness and cruelty that you didn't expect. Sometimes those who suffer social pain the most are those who are the most idealistic. Strive to hold on to both sides: aware of both the greatness and the awfulness that human beings are capable of.

Learn how others cope. Search online using terms such as *overcoming stigma, how to cope with discrimination, what to do about scapegoating,* etc.

Notice whether you keep replaying certain conversations in your mind. You may have repeated revenge fantasies or feel stuck in other ways (see "Dark feelings: Rage, hatred, revenge, bitterness," Chapter 29).

As you gain solid recovery, social pain goes down. Recovery offers experiences that are different from the past, like new branches on a tree.

✧ Do you have at least one person you can truly open up to about social pain? If not, how can you try to start finding that?

✧ Are there any suggestions you can try from the section called *What to do about it?*

RECOVERY VOICES

Jennyfer – " . . . a buffer that shields me"

At 15, Jennyfer was hit by a stray bullet, resulting in traumatic brain injury, PTSD, and drug abuse as a way to cope. "That one moment of being shot has defined me in so many ways. It's changed my view of myself, although that's something I can work on. How others respond to me is much harder. Even strangers – I can't tell you how many times complete strangers ask me, 'Why do you walk like that? Were you in a car accident? Do you have multiple sclerosis?' It also creates anxiety – forming new relationships is difficult, as I feel I need to explain a huge event from my past without its somehow defining me; and it opens up the possibility of others rejecting me because of something I had no control over. Previous rejections pile on top of each other and create an emotional scar that makes me averse to being vulnerable, which is a major obstacle to intimacy and closeness. I see social pain in others too; it's not just my own experience. There's so much shame and stigma with trauma. War veterans and others who suffered traumatic brain injury are labeled as crazy or weird. Those who are sexually assaulted are assumed to be promiscuous or 'asked for it' because of how they acted or dressed. This stuff still happens *a lot*. What I appreciate about this chapter is that it gives language to these experiences. When there's social pain on top of trauma and addiction, it adds a layer of struggle that makes it that much harder to recover. There's that well-worn phrase 'If you walked a mile in my shoes. . . . ' What's

needed more are people who can hear what it's really like to live with these problems, trying to recover from them. Sometimes I get angry at people's cluelessness
and lack of empathy. But then I remind myself that there are also amazing people
out there who do get it or at least want to. I try to surround myself with those
people and, more than anything else, that helps me lessen the social pain. It's a
buffer that shields me from the ones who don't get it."

14

True self-compassion

If you want others to be happy, practice compassion. If you want to be happy, practice compassion.

—DALAI LAMA XIV, Tibetan leader and winner of the Nobel Peace Prize

Compassion allows you to stop blaming yourself and instead *understand* yourself. But it's not a simplistic view of compassion. The ultimate test of compassion is whether it helps you change unhealthy behavior. Compassion without behavior change means it's not deep enough.

True compassion can be powerful. Many people believe compassion is weakness – just making excuses or letting yourself off the hook – but it's not. You may be surprised to hear that greater compassion toward yourself leads to stronger motivation to change, according to research.

An Example of Compassion Toward Yourself

An example of self-compassion might go like this:

> "I really want that drink, but with my family's history of alcoholism I know it's not safe for me. My friends can drink, but I can't. It's totally unfair, but I have to accept it. Maybe I can give myself some other treat that's safe. With all the horrible trauma I've lived through, I want to be kind to myself as I go through this."

Notice how this example:

» Is gentle and encouraging ("I want to be kind to myself")

» Is realistic about what's safe and unsafe ("I know it's not safe for me"; "My friends can drink, but I can't")

» Offers a broad perspective ("my family history of alcoholism," "with all the trauma I've lived through")

» Identifies a new path ("give myself some other treat")

» Accepts reality ("I have to accept it")

◇ Do you notice a softer heart after reading this? If not, that's okay, keep reading . . .

If you received little compassion in the past, it may be hard to understand until you start doing it. It may feel uncomfortable at first, but eventually you'll find it's essential for healthy living.

True Compassion

Compassion is not just cheerleading or saying positive things to yourself. It's not just being nice or feeling good. Recovery requires you to sacrifice and deprive yourself at times. Turning down a drink is tough when you're craving it. Leaving a partner who hurts you may feel wrong but you know it's right. Psychologist Marsha Linehan calls this *wise mind*: doing what you know is right. Compassion is not about the easy choice, the one that feels best; it's about doing what *is* best.

Kristin Neff, a psychologist who studies compassion, writes, ". . . having compassion for oneself entails desiring health and well-being for oneself, which means gently encouraging change where needed and rectifying harmful or unproductive patterns of behavior. Thus, self-compassion should counteract complacency."

What Compassion Is Not

It's also useful to understand what compassion *isn't*. It isn't about:

» Making excuses

» Justifying bad choices

» Letting yourself off the hook for mistakes

» Whitewashing the truth

» Pretending all is fine ("rose-colored glasses")

» Arrogance ("I'm always right")

» Selfishness

» Pity

You may make bad choices at times even if they're not always your fault. You may spend time with unsafe people, ignore tasks at work or home, drive under the influence, and so on. Your addiction and trauma problems may have led you to behaviors that harm you and others.

Charles was addicted to methamphetamine. "My brother Sean was killed by a drug dealer who mistook Sean for me. My choices cost him his life; I can't forgive myself."

Compassion means you own your mistakes and strive to understand them, taking a wide-angle view to what got you there. The more you do this, the better you become at not repeating them. You gain understanding rather than judgment.

How to decide if compassion is working? Watch your behavior – it is your compass and your truest guide. True compassion is when you're gentler with yourself, yet more responsible. You have less addictive behavior, you take better care of your body, you follow through on commitments. See "Listen to your behavior," Chapter 7, for more.

Compassion toward Yourself

It's easier to be compassionate toward others than toward yourself. This is true for most people, but especially so if you have addiction and trauma problems. You may believe that being hard on yourself is normal or necessary. If you were treated badly, you may have learned to hate rather than encourage yourself. Or some people have the opposite problem – they're arrogant, believing they're always right. But overhating and overloving yourself are flip sides of each other. People with a healthy sense of self are aware of their strengths and weaknesses in a balanced way.

Real change happens when you balance *love* and *limits* – warm support plus firm accountability. If you're too easy or too hard on yourself, you stay stuck. You may also be bouncing between these, caught up in a cycle of too much indulgence/too much harshness. You feel bad, so you gamble too much and then beat yourself up for it, which makes you more likely to gamble again, and the cycle continues.

Ashley said, "Inside my head is constant self-hatred. 'I'm a loser,' 'I'm fat,' 'I'll never amount to anything.' To turn off that voice I binge and purge, but it never gets rid of the self-loathing."

It's never too late to learn compassion. It can become a powerful presence, like a caring friend who is supportive but also doesn't let you get away with things.

✧ Try talking to yourself with compassion right now even if it feels hard to do.

Compassion toward Others

Compassion toward others can also be healing and can strengthen your recovery (see "What the wounded can give back," Chapter 34). But you never have to take a compassionate view toward people who harmed you. If you want to develop compassion for them, you can, but it's a choice, not a requirement – you can recover without it.

If you decide to do it, keep it healthy. Codependency (addiction to a person, loosely speaking) or severe relationship trauma can leave you without healthy boundaries. You may go overboard with love-at-any-cost "compassion" – unbalanced, too tolerant, enabling. You may offer compassion to people who keep betraying you. In good relationships, both people give and receive and have each other's interests at heart.

Know, too, that compassion and forgiveness aren't the same. You can have compassion for people without forgiving them. You may understand why someone harmed you, how it was rooted in pain or their own trauma – but that doesn't mean you have to forgive. You don't have to forgive to heal (see "Forgiving yourself," Chapter 16).

⋆ Explore . . . *How do you score on compassion?*

Self-Compassion

Take the Self-Compassion Scale (*www.self-compassion.org/test-how-self-compassionate-you-are*). It's a free, valid scale you can do anonymously online to see how compassionate you are toward yourself. It includes questions like these:

- "I try to be loving toward myself when I'm feeling emotional pain."
- "When I fail at something important to me, I try to keep things in perspective."

- "I try to be understanding and patient toward those aspects of my personality I don't like."

- "I try to see my failings as part of the human condition."

- "When I feel inadequate in some way, I try to remind myself that feelings of inadequacy are shared by most people."

Compassion for Others

You can also see how you score on compassion toward others. Go to *http://self-compassion.org/self-compassion-scales-for-researchers* to find the Compassion for Others Scale. It includes questions such as these:

- "I notice when people are upset, even if they don't say anything."

- "I like to be there for others in times of difficulty."

- "When others feel sadness, I try to comfort them."

- "Everyone feels down sometimes; it's part of being human."

- "It's important to recognize that all people have weaknesses and no one's perfect."

✧ How did you score? What do the scores reveal about you?

✧ What does *true compassion* mean?

✧ Can you be kind to yourself yet still work really hard on recovery?

RECOVERY VOICES

David – "Changing the lens to compassion is beautiful."

"This is my favorite chapter. I use it to define compassion through my eyes. When using drugs and engaging in trauma reenactments, I beat myself up physically and mentally. Would I do that to a friend? No way. Would I treat a child the way I sometimes treat myself? No way. So using this chapter to take a look at my worldview and change the lens to one of compassion was beautiful. Active addiction and trauma symptoms means a very cold, angry, scared experience. Compassion cuts through all that, but it definitely takes practice to be compassionate.

I could take the messages I'd noted in "Every child is a detective" [Chapter 22] and look for opportunities in my day to practice either embracing them if they were compassionate, or challenging them if they were not. I think to get good at anything you need to practice, and since my default is to be harsh with myself I have many opportunities to practice throughout my day. I could also keep track of my feelings and behaviors throughout my compassionate practice. My actions don't lie, so if I find that by practicing compassion with myself and others I see an increase in the previously identified positive activities, I know compassion has benefit. I will need to challenge myself to practice compassion because it's hard to do. I will remind myself throughout the day that I'm striving to have a compassionate mind-set. I will keep a list of compassionate statements with me so that I can remind myself of the direction I want to go."

15

⸙

Why trauma and addiction go together

What one understands is only half true. What one does not understand is the full truth.
—Zen saying

Trauma and addiction have been called *brother and sister maladies* because they so often go together. They're part of the same family. Yet even people who have suffered both for many years often don't see the connection between them.

Alex: "I never put it together before – how my drinking came out of what I went through as a kid. Now it makes sense. I don't feel so ashamed anymore. I can work on it now."

It's Not about the *Thing* (the Substance, the Food, the Sex)

People usually think that addiction occurs because something "is addictive," such as alcohol, gambling, or pornography. But most people who try these don't get addicted to them. So it's not the thing itself; it's the person + the thing = addiction. Of course, some things are more likely to become addictive than others; cocaine is more addictive than spinach. But just as what's traumatic for one person may not be for another, what's addictive for one person may not be for another. Even a given person may be vulnerable to addiction at one time but not another, depending on the circumstances. So throughout your life you need to carefully watch the impact of *your* activities on *your* life.

Numbing the Pain: How Trauma Makes People Vulnerable to Addiction

One big reason some people develop addiction is that they've lived through serious trauma. It's been called *deadly logic*: it makes sense to reach out for something to try to feel better. It's also called *self-medication, numbing the pain,* or *using to escape.* The addictive behavior feels like a solution for trauma problems, at least for a while. Some people with severe trauma and addiction say they made a decision to keep using because it was the only way they could get relief from emotional pain. Other vulnerabilities add to the impact as well, such as homelessness, poverty, mental health problems, discrimination, and social isolation.

Marco grew up in a war-torn country where violence was a constant threat. He felt tense and afraid much of the time. He said, "I was 12 when I tried my first drink and knew immediately this was my solution. I felt more relaxed than I'd ever felt before."

Stacy was abused as a child. "When you're being terrorized at home and you discover a substance, it's like, 'This is it. This is the only thing that brings some relief.' Even though you know it's temporary and it can destroy your life, it feels like your life is already destroyed anyway. There's nothing worth saving, so it's six of one, half-dozen of another."

Paul's mother was mentally ill and verbally abusive. When he discovered opiates, "It was like from heaven, like love at first sight . . . I could feel at peace, more loving . . . more lovable."

—Adapted from *Understanding Addiction as Self-Medication: Finding Hope behind the Pain* by Edward Khantzian and Mark Albanese

---

The deadly logic is shown by research too. People with trauma problems, compared to those without trauma problems:

» Start using substances earlier

» Have more positive views of substances

» Move more quickly from substance use to addiction

» Have more relapses

» Use hard drugs more, such as cocaine, opiates, and methamphetamine

» Are less likely to stop using even once they're in treatment for addiction

Yet it can take years to see the connection between trauma and addiction. Often, the addiction is visible first and the trauma history is recognized only later.

Self-Protection

Some people say that addictive behavior allowed them to survive trauma they couldn't escape. It numbed them out so they wouldn't commit suicide. It was their only friend when they were isolated in trauma. It was a brief escape from a brutal reality.

Marissa was married to a man with serious addiction and domestic violence problems. She said, "I drank all day, every day, and didn't stop till I blacked out. I think it was my way of dealing with my husband. My children basically raised themselves, took care of themselves, fed themselves, and took care of me. As his addiction got worse and the beatings got worse, I got worse. There'd be times when I'd wake up not able to move, and I wouldn't even remember what had happened. And my 8-year-old son would have to tell me how Daddy had beat me the night before. I'd go to work drunk. I just lived drunk, was how I dealt with it all."
—Adapted from *Example of a Group Session: Asking for Help (Seeking Safety* video training, by Lisa M. Najavits)

Some Subgroups Are More Likely to Develop Trauma and Addiction

People with trauma and addiction are of all ages, ethnicities, social classes, gender orientations, and educational backgrounds. But some subgroups are especially vulnerable to trauma and addiction, including:

- » Military and veterans
- » Adolescents
- » Domestic violence victims
- » Homeless
- » Elderly
- » Physically or mentally disabled
- » Lesbian, gay, bisexual, transgendered

» Criminal justice populations

» Sex workers

» Some ethnic groups

» War refugees

» First responders such as firefighters, police, and emergency workers

These subgroups are at heightened risk for trauma and thus vulnerable to addiction too. For example, senior citizens may suffer elder abuse and are at risk for addictions such as gambling and misuse of prescription medications. Adolescents are at an age where sexual assault and violence may be occurring at the same time as experimentation with substances, gambling, and other addictive behavior. Military personnel and first responders have heightened rates of trauma and may be given painkiller medication to treat injuries, which can become addictive.

Don is a Vietnam veteran. "After I came back from war, I was a completely changed person who could not take orders or direction from anyone. I was extremely restless and became bored easily. . . . I was angry about everything and thought that the government did whatever it wanted to do and so could I . . . I smoked a lot of pot, which I had learned to use in Vietnam. None of my friends used [drugs] before I went overseas, and neither did I. After 'Nam there wasn't a drug I wouldn't smoke, swallow, or snort. The alcohol and substance abuse was fueled by my need to forget the things that kept me up at night and to fire my addiction to adrenaline. In a war zone, adrenaline is your friend. My disruptive behavior got worse year by year. I needed more excitement to fill the void that 'normal life' left in me. I did not understand the changes in me and didn't really care as long as I could get the excitement I craved."
—From *The Warzone PTSD Survivors Guide*, by Donald G. Parent, Jr.

Various Pathways

If you have both trauma and addiction, how did they arise? Awareness of your life patterns can deepen your recovery.

Trauma occurs first, then addiction. This is the most common pattern, for about two-thirds of people. It's often called *self-medication*: trying to feel better through behavior that eventually becomes addictive. For example, a man is distraught over his son's death and begins abusing prescription painkillers.

Addiction occurs first, then trauma. This pattern is called *vulnerability*: the addiction makes trauma more likely. For example, an alcoholic drives drunk and gets into an accident, or a sex addict is assaulted when engaging in a hookup.

Both arise together. For some people trauma and addiction occur at the same time. Children may grow up in families where trauma is ever-present and so is addiction. In fact, one of the biggest predictors of both addiction and trauma problems is family history. They repeat across generations based on both genes and social factors (see "Body and biology," Chapter 17, and "Every child is a detective," Chapter 22, for more).

Each arises on its own. Although not common, some people develop unrelated trauma and addiction problems, just as a person can develop two unrelated medical conditions such as diabetes and cancer. For example, Carmen is elderly and has had a drinking problem for years; recently she developed PTSD from a fire at her nursing home. In her case, the two problems arose separately.

Downward Spirals and Upward Spirals

Trauma and addiction feed off each other in what's called a *downward spiral* or *toxic feedback loop*. It's stress upon stress, damage on damage, over and over. Trauma leads to addiction, which leads to more trauma, which leads to more addiction. Or addiction leads to trauma, which leads to more addiction. They reinforce each other, deepening their hold on you. But remember: just as trauma and addiction problems are linked, so is their recovery. Improving one can help the other in an *upward spiral*.

Become a Detective

If you have both addiction and trauma problems, watch how they impact each other in the present too. All combinations are possible. Addiction use, withdrawal, or abstinence can make your trauma problems better or worse. So, too, both trauma problems and trauma recovery can make your addiction better or worse. Some people find, for example, that after months or years of abstinence from substances their trauma problems flare up – they notice feelings and memories they had been pushing away with substances. Others find their trauma problems get better – they are handling all of their issues with greater strength and coping. There is no one pattern, so just stay aware of yours. Over time, you can gain solid recovery from both.

Many Reasons for Using – Not Just Trauma

People have addictive behavior for many different reasons; it's not always about trauma. It can be to:

» Celebrate

» Seek thrills

» Have fun

» Gain insight

» Relax

» Connect with others

» Enhance a feeling

» Be more sexual

» Feel more energy

Intoxication – the search for transcendent pleasure – is a basic human drive. People want to feel good and to have out-of-the-ordinary experiences. Since earliest human history, substance use, usually alcohol, has been part of most societies. Some cultural traditions have rituals to induce transcendent states through rhythmic drumming or dancing. Like sex, food, play, and other pleasurable experiences, intoxication is a regular part of life for many people. They have a drink with dinner or gamble a small amount of money and then go on with their lives. They have enough fulfilling experiences that they don't need to keep using. The intoxication doesn't interfere with their responsibilities or cause serious harm. They're not using it to escape intense sadness, emptiness, or loneliness.

Other people start to develop a problem but cut back on their own. They have *natural recovery* – they stop or reduce their use when they notice negative consequences from it. In fact, most people who develop mild alcohol problems (*problem drinkers*) recover on their own, especially if they catch the problem early. And some people use too much during a phase of their lives, such as drinking too much in college, but after that they mature and move on.

For others, however, intoxication becomes an unhealthy obsession. Trauma is often part of that pattern.

⋆ Explore . . . *Your patterns of trauma, addiction, or both*

There are no right or wrong answers to these questions. The goal is awareness.

1. Which arose first for you?

   a. Trauma

   b. Addiction

   c. Both at the same time

   d. I don't have problems with both

   e. I'm not sure

Explore your answer. For most people with both trauma and addiction, the trauma occurred first. But whichever came first, if you have problems with both you need to work on both. If you have just one – trauma problems or addiction – your recovery may go more quickly than if you had both.

2. Which are you more motivated to work on?

   a. Trauma

   b. Addiction

   c. Both equally

   d. Neither

   e. I don't have problems with both

   f. I'm not sure

Explore your answer. If you have both addiction and trauma problems, it's common to feel more motivated to work on one than the other. Usually, trauma problems are more motivating because they create direct emotional pain, such as depression, nightmares, and flashbacks. Addiction causes suffering too, but it may take longer to see it, as denial is often part of the illness. Whichever you feel more motivated to work on, use that as a starting point; it can increase motivation to work on the other too. This is called *leveraging* one problem to help the other. For example, "I have trauma nightmares, and cocaine makes them worse, so I need to stop using cocaine." If you don't feel motivation to work on either one, know that motivation increases the more you keep learning and exploring.

3. Which is a greater problem for you right now?

    a. Trauma

    b. Addiction

    c. Both equally

    d. Neither is a problem

    e. I'm not sure

Explore your answer. Some people have more problems from one than the other. Just keep noticing how they show up for you.

4. Which is part of your family history (at least one relative)?

    a. Trauma

    b. Addiction

    c. Both

    d. Neither

    e. I'm not sure

    If you marked a, b, or c: How many relatives (approximately)? _____

Explore your answer. Family history is one of the biggest predictors of trauma and addiction: both run in families. Genes and social influences play a role, which is why the question does not focus just on blood relatives. If you have a family history of trauma problems, addiction, or both, know that family history isn't a "life sentence." It's all about how you respond to that history. The earlier and stronger your recovery efforts, the more likely you are to prevent these issues from continuing into the next generation. It can be a point of great pride to stop the cycle.

5. My addiction generally makes my trauma problems

    a. Worse

    b. Better

    c. No different

    d. It depends – sometimes worse, sometimes better

    e. Not applicable (no addictive behavior)

    f. I'm not sure

Now re-ask yourself this question in reverse: "My trauma problems generally make my addiction . . . "

Explore your answer. Notice how your addiction and trauma problems impact each other if you have both. And know that you can learn to respond successfully to both.

❖ Do you notice any new insights from reading this chapter?

❖ If you have both trauma and addiction problems, how are they linked – in your life and in your family history?

RECOVERY VOICES

David – "Being a detective"

"I use this chapter to help me understand how my trauma is intertwined with my addictions. I like the very simple questions to explore my patterns because often my head feels foggy and I have difficulty seeing how my experiences drive my behaviors. This chapter also makes me feel like I was kind of being a detective. What I noticed is that almost every time I used drugs I engaged in severe reenactments of my trauma, and then I experienced more trauma by placing myself in unsafe situations to obtain more drugs and 'act out' my trauma. This chapter helped me understand my actions and bizarre behaviors so I feel less like a freak and more compassionate with myself. It clarified what was impacting me the most between drugs and trauma. The trauma was painful, but my drug use was putting me at risk for violence and incredible self-harm. Both were pretty bad, though. I take this information and use it to refine my recovery program and guide me with next steps."

16

Forgiving yourself

> Forgiveness is the answer to the child's dream . . . what is broken is made whole again.
>
> —DAG HAMMARSKJÖLD, 20th-century Swedish diplomat and winner of the Nobel Peace Prize

Forgiving yourself is a challenging task of recovery. You may need to forgive yourself for:

- What you did ▪ What you didn't do ▪ Who you hurt ▪ How you reacted during trauma ▪ Surviving when others didn't ▪ Crimes you committed ▪ Failing your children or family ▪ What you did to your body ▪ What you didn't know ▪ Bad judgment ▪ Poor decisions ▪ Feelings you're ashamed of ▪ How your body responded ▪ Addiction problems ▪ Trauma problems ▪ Not measuring up ▪ Wasting time ▪ What you lost

✧ What do you have difficulty forgiving yourself for?

Trauma and addiction often lead to shame, guilt, self-blame, and self-hatred. If life has been too hard or you were treated badly, it's human nature to turn against yourself.

Forgiving yourself means coming to terms with what happened and doing your best to make the future better than the past. It doesn't mean you like what happened, that it was right, or that you would make the same choices again. It doesn't mean you forgive others for what they did to you. It only means that you make peace with your part in what happened. It's letting go of the resentments toward yourself, knowing that even if flawed, you can respect that you were who you were at the time and you always have the capacity to grow going forward.

How

Discover new truths. You can arrive at insights that help you release yourself:

» "No one taught me differently, so I didn't know."

» "I made some bad choices, but I also made good ones."

» "I was influenced by people that I won't ever let influence me again."

» "I've learned and can make other choices next time."

» "I'm imperfect just like everyone else."

» "No matter what I did in the past I can be different now."

» "I survived an awful situation; there were no good choices available."

» "I was alone and did the best I could to figure it out."

» "It's within my power to forgive myself."

» "Even if others won't forgive me, I can forgive myself."

» "I felt so low that I didn't have it in me to try harder."

» "I did what I thought was best at the time, even if I see it differently now."

» "There are many reasons for what happened (genetics, family history, culture, lack of support, etc.) – not just some flaw in me."

» "I wish I could have controlled what happened, but I couldn't."

» "I'm still alive and I get to try again."

Feel the forgiveness. Try to let yourself *feel* the forgiveness. It's a sort of letting go, relaxing into acceptance of what you did or didn't do. You may need to search your heart for the part of you, even if small, that takes your side of the inner debate, that allies with the most vulnerable sides of you. Forgiveness feels like you're there for yourself, not in a false way ("I'm always right"), but in a quiet way that accepts the full truth of what happened. Letting yourself feel the forgiveness may be painful at first, but the pain melts into larger awareness.

Channel yourself toward helping others. It can also help to face forward and contribute to any type of mission that allows you to offer something good to the world to try to make up for what you feel you did wrong. Try to pick something meaningful for you. For example, you might volunteer to help other veterans in memory of the buddy you couldn't save during war. But if you take this approach, stay focused on healthy balance – not letting atonement become so extreme that you lose your sense of self and your own life goals.

Apologize. If you hurt others in the past and that plays a role in your difficulty forgiving yourself, you can apologize if it's safe to do so. The AA process of *making amends* provides an excellent example of that for addiction.

See also "True self-compassion" (Chapter 14), which describes how to take a kind view of yourself while still holding yourself accountable.

Is It Necessary to Forgive Others?

Forgiving others is an option, never a requirement. And you never have to forgive someone who hurt you unless you arrive at that in a genuine way. It can't be forced, and it's *not* necessary for healing despite what people may tell you. Indeed, it can be damaging to be pushed into forgiveness that you don't feel. It's a personal choice and it may take years or decades to decide whether you want to forgive people who hurt you. Forgiving others is not the goal or the endpoint of the work you're doing within yourself. If it happens, it happens; if not, you can still heal.

In the trauma field, it's well established that forgiveness is a choice, not a requirement. In the addiction field, you're more likely to hear that you must forgive, but that idea developed before the addiction field focused on trauma. Now the idea is that forgiveness is always a personal choice. You can make progress with or without it.

But forgiving *yourself* is key. Otherwise, there may be some part of the past always holding you back.

✶ Explore . . . *Self-forgiveness*

Try either or both of these exercises.

Exercise 1: *Imagine Being Forgiven by Someone You Respect*

a) Think of someone you know who cares about you and is also genuinely good – it might be a parent, friend, teacher, mentor, spiritual advisor, or a higher power.

b) Now explore an imaginary conversation with that person about your difficulty forgiving yourself. What would you say to that person? What would the person say to you? What would you want to hear from the person? What feelings would they convey toward you?

Exercise 2: *Write about It*

Read the following quotation. Write about it with as much kindness toward yourself as possible.

> ". . . forgiveness is giving up all hope of having had a different past."
> —From *Traveling Mercies* by Anne Lamott

✧ What do you want to forgive yourself for?

✧ How can self-forgiveness help your recovery?

RECOVERY VOICES

Bridget – "I was carrying a lock in my heart."

"I'm a survivor of child sexual and emotional abuse. I've been addicted to food, spending, relationships, and emotional chaos. Self-forgiveness has been the hardest part of my recovery. It's also the last piece I've put into place. What I'd say to somebody else is, know that you can do this; it can happen. But you really have to open your heart. And it may happen in such small steps that it's hard to feel it. One thing I like about this chapter is how it says you need to let yourself *feel* the forgiveness; that's the hardest part. I got it intellectually a whole lot sooner than I got it emotionally. I could feel it toward other people – I was a great caretaker – but I couldn't feel it for myself. I tried a lot of things – religion, affirmations, positive psychology. I tried that exercise where you imagine how you'd talk kindly to a young child. I even tried to channel myself toward social change to help others, and that was a good thing, but it didn't get to the bottom line, which is can I sit with myself? Can I be here with me? I know that when I draw that last breath, I want to be okay with me.

"My dad was vicious. He was a working-class drunk – the devaluing, beating-you-down stuff. The thing I really relate to in other trauma survivors is the self-hatred, the total venom toward myself, like I don't have enough worth to be on the planet. And with addiction, no matter what type it is, whether it's alcohol, drugs, or any other behavior, you feel like people can always point a finger and say, 'Well, you're doing it to yourself.' There's so much stigma and blame, and you internalize that and think, 'Yes, I'm the problem here.' So the starting point for me was just to be *aware* of the negativity I was perpetrating on myself. And what I tell other people and what I try to remember myself is that it's never too late to get out of hell. It's never too late. No matter what age you are, even if you're 80 years old, you can still get to the peace that comes with self-forgiveness and that's so enormous.

"The breakthrough for me was when I was sitting looking out the window at a beautiful redwood tree and I thought, 'Oh my god, I've spent my entire adult life (and that's a long time at this point) as a substance abuse counselor helping addicts recognize that they *deserved* forgiveness. I could always see their goodness, but I couldn't see my own. It was always, 'Yeah, but . . . yeah, but" toward myself. And I finally said, 'Wait a minute – I've helped so many people with this; why am I different? The things I blame myself for doing, why don't I ever let myself off the hook?' I was carrying a lock in my heart. But then I got it – and it's different for everyone what tips the balance – but for me it was that I realized that I had spent 30 years giving other people permission to forgive themselves but I hadn't given that to myself. I had worked with people who had done some really awful things, like kill people. I worked in addiction and heard awful stories. So somehow that's when I really got it for myself. There's a sadness to this – grieving about the time you lost, the things you've done and maybe that other people won't forgive you. But you really need to get that whether they forgive you or not is not the point. It's whether you forgive you. And the other thing that's really important to get is that it's not about forgiving other people. Maybe you will and maybe you won't. The point is you forgive yourself because until you forgive yourself you're still trapped – and that's the destruction of a life."

17

Body and biology

The body says what words cannot.
—MARTHA GRAHAM, 20th-century choreographer
and winner of the Presidential Medal of Freedom

What story does your body tell? What roles do trauma and addiction play in that story? This chapter explores those questions – linking past and present, body and mind.

Trauma and Addiction Are Physical in Nature

Trauma and addiction are experienced *in the body*. Many traumas are physical events, such as physical and sexual abuse, car accidents, hurricanes, serious medical illnesses, combat, and fires. Emotional abuse takes a toll on the body too.

Addictions are rooted in physical excesses – drinking too much alcohol, taking drugs, excessive food, sex, pornography, shopping, tanning, exercise, and self-harm such as cutting. Even addictions that don't seem physical, such as gambling, show brain patterns similar to those for substance addiction. And addictive behavior is sometimes used to manage physical problems – to cope with physical illness or injury; to lose weight; to sleep; to manage body changes related to adolescence or aging.

What does all this mean? It means you need to pay strong attention to your body as part of recovery. You may need to "hear" your body more – noticing when you feel pain or discomfort rather than ignoring it. It may mean making more effort to take care of your body, such as eating healthily and getting exercise. It may involve forging a new relationship with your body based on respecting it. No matter how much trauma or addiction you've had, you can learn to live in harmony with your body.

This chapter was adapted with permission from *Creating Change* by Lisa M. Najavits (forthcoming from The Guilford Press).

Biology Matters – But Is Not Destiny

The sections that follow describe physical vulnerabilities you may have from trauma and addiction. But they are not a life sentence. With recovery, the brain and body improve too.

In Conflict with Your Body

You may hate your body or parts of it. You may resent physical reminders of addiction such as needle marks. You may be upset about what your body did during trauma, such as sexual arousal during rape or freezing rather than fighting. You may have put on weight ("soft armor") in response to unwanted sexual attention. You may have distorted perceptions about how your body looks to others.

As a teen, Brian was sexually assaulted by a family "friend" during a beach weekend. "No matter how many showers I took that night I felt dirty. When I went to a family picnic the next day I was sure they could tell what had happened to me – that they just knew by looking at me. I drank a lot, sneaking so many beers that I threw up. They couldn't figure out what that was about, and I couldn't tell them."

Your Body Speaking for You

Your body may express physically what you haven't dealt with emotionally. You may have nausea or headaches when you remember trauma. Some people even become blind or mute after severe trauma, but there's no known physical cause. Others report *body memories* from trauma, such as feeling as if they can't breathe – like flashbacks, but instead of visual images they are physical sensations. As you work on trauma and addiction, learning to express what you feel inside, your physical problems may improve.

✦ Do you notice any physical problems that are based in emotional pain?

Unaware of Your Body

Trauma and addiction can decrease body awareness. You may feel numb, not notice physical problems (ignoring a toothache or broken bone), or not attend to hunger or thirst. You may *dissociate,* which means that your mind detaches for a while in response to stress; during these times, you may feel unaware of body sensations.

Medical Care Challenges

People with trauma and addiction have greater distrust of medical staff and worse follow-through on medical advice (not getting necessary tests, not taking medications as prescribed). For other people, trauma and addiction lead to much higher use of medical care than the average person, such as more emergency room visits.

Sexual Problems

Some sexual problems relate to trauma and addiction: feeling triggered during sex, having unsafe sex, exchanging sex for drugs, becoming addicted to sex or porn, and hooking up with dangerous people. Sex can also *reenact* (repeat) trauma themes that you experienced. Or you may have fear of sex, lack of sexual feelings, and difficulty being intimate. Some people use substances to be able to engage in sex.

Physical Problems

Trauma and addiction wear down the body. People with trauma and addiction have more physical problems than others, including heart and stomach problems, sexually transmitted diseases, low energy, headaches, joint pain, liver disease, bone fractures, less ability to fight infection, HIV, chronic pain, hepatitis, and worse pregnancy outcomes. And some physical conditions are immediate results of trauma or addiction – being hit can cause brain damage; cocaine use can trigger a heart attack. In a major study of more than 10,000 people, the more that children were exposed to trauma and addiction in their family, the worse their physical health was later in life (*www.acestudy.org*).

Giving Up on Your Body

Trauma and addiction may bring you so low that you don't care what happens to your body. You may share unclean needles, have unsafe sex, or not take care of yourself during pregnancy. You may neglect medical and dental care.

Jamie served 2 years in Iraq. "I didn't die over there, but I died inside. What we had to do to innocent people – families, kids – made me sick. It hardened my soul. I have images I'll live with for the rest of my life. I used to be fit, but I stopped caring. I'm 50 pounds overweight and have prediabetes. I smoke and drink too much. I'm 38 and feel like I'm in an older man's body."

Sensitivity to Physical Pain

People with a history of trauma perceive pain more intensely than people without that history. Some addictions, such as opiate abuse, also create hypersensitivity to pain.

Brain Changes

The brain is a physical part of your body as much as your arms and legs. To see how different substances affect the brain, you can search for *brain scans substance abuse*. The good news is that, with abstinence from substances, the brain heals and looks normal again, according to the National Institute on Drug Abuse (2014). Neglect or repeated abuse in childhood affects brain development too, and the more often it occurs, the greater the impact. Both trauma and addiction degrade mental processes such as concentration, attention, memory, planning, judgment, reasoning, and flexibility (you may find yourself getting stuck going over the same things in your mind). They're also associated with *traumatic brain injury* (TBI), which can occur when the head is injured, such as in car accidents or military combat. Whatever brain changes you've had, know that new learning can offset damage that occurred due to trauma, addiction, or TBI. New experiences can rewire the brain in healthy directions.

Triggering

Triggers are quick, intense negative reactions, both physical and emotional. It's your body's way of trying to protect you. You may find yourself reacting to trauma triggers such as sudden sounds, darkness, certain foods, or places. You may be on high alert and easily startled. Your body learned that some things are unsafe and now reacts before you're even aware of it. Studies of PTSD show that even after years of recovery such automatic reactions often persist. But even if your body's instinct is to react, you can gain control over your behavior.

Addiction creates triggering too. People, places, or things that remind you of using set off a cascade of physical reactions that makes the behavior hard to resist. Research shows that your brain responds even before you're aware of the craving. But the longer you're in recovery, the less intense the triggering.

> ✧ What are your trauma triggers? Addiction triggers? How can you protect yourself from them?

Stress

Stress means your body and mind are overwhelmed. It's a physical response in humans and animals that promotes survival. When you face danger your muscles tense, you breathe faster, your brain uses more oxygen so it can process more information – all to help you face a threat and take the best course of action (flight, fight, or freeze). In the short term, stress helps you, but if it's ongoing your body gets worn out by being on high alert for long periods of time. After a while it has trouble returning to a normal state. Ongoing stress leads to physical and emotional problems. Stress is also the leading cause of addiction relapse, according to the National Institute on Drug Abuse. And stress is part of the very term "posttraumatic *stress* disorder." Try to reduce stress wherever possible. Some people have felt stressed for so long that they forget what calm actually feels like.

✧ What can you do *today* to decrease stress?

Family Vulnerability

Addiction and trauma problems run in families, partly based on genes – inherited from your biological "blood" relatives. Just as eye color and height are based on genes, so are many medical illnesses, including vulnerability to PTSD and substance abuse (the most studied addiction). This doesn't mean you're doomed to them, but you may be more likely to develop them and may have to work harder to overcome them if they run in your family. It also means it's important to try to protect your children from developing them.

✫ Explore . . . *Your relationship with your body*

Circle one answer in each row in the table on the next page, thinking about the past 3 months. Use the words in the top row to guide your answers: *not at all/a little/moderately/a lot*. Don't focus on the numbers, as some rows have the numbers reversed for scoring purposes.

Your Relationship with Your Body

	Not at all	A little	Moder- ately	A lot
1. Are you physically healthy?	0	1	2	3
2. Do you take good care of your body?	0	1	2	3
3. Do you feel positive about sex?	0	1	2	3
4. Do you have any current physically oriented addictions (e.g., substances, food, shopping, sex, tanning, surgery, exercise)?	3	2	1	0
5. How much stress do you have in your life?	3	2	1	0
6. Is anyone, including you, directly harming your body (e.g., self-harm, domestic violence)?	3	2	1	0
7. How safe do you feel in your body?	0	1	2	3
8. When you look in the mirror, do you feel positive about your body (body image)?	0	1	2	3
9. Do you pursue high-risk physical activities (e.g., unsafe sex, dangerous sports, reckless driving, driving under the influence)?	3	2	1	0
10. Do you feel comfortable being touched by someone you like?	0	1	2	3
11. How aware are you of your body (its "moods," sensations, changes)?	0	1	2	3
12. Do you get necessary medical care (doctors and dentists, following up on their advice, etc.)?	0	1	2	3

13. Do you have any current medical conditions that affect your body in an ongoing way (e.g., chronic pain, diabetes, cancer, traumatic brain injury)?	3	2	1	0
14. Do you have any current mental health conditions that affect your body in an ongoing way (e.g., eating disorder, hair-pulling, skin picking)?	3	2	1	0
15. Do you ignore body pain or injury that you need to attend to?	3	2	1	0
16. How much do you appreciate your body, even with its flaws?	0	1	2	3

Scoring: Add up the numbers you circled. What is your total? _____ The closer your number is to 48, the more positive your relationship with your body.

✧ If your body could speak, what would it say?

✧ Are there any medical appointments you need to make? Can you call right now?

✧ If you viewed your body as your best friend, what would you do differently?

✧ Do you remember what it feels like for your body to be truly calm?

✧ How can you put in place healthier eating, exercise, and sleep?

RECOVERY VOICES

Katrina – "Symptoms were my body crying out for help."

Katrina is an Army veteran who experienced physical, sexual, and emotional trauma during her service. "While on active duty I worked in electronics and unit armor. I suffered a major injury in a shop accident that caused me to become unfit for duty, although that wasn't officially recognized at first. So I kept working for 5 years until my body could no longer take it, and then I was out of work the next 10 years, disabled. I couldn't dress myself, couldn't shower myself. It just hadn't kicked in right away how bad it was – I was like, 'I'll just suck it up.' I had suppressed all my pain and symptoms the way I was trained to. I soldiered on until that was no longer possible, until I collapsed. The attitude in the military toward physical complaints was that weakness is a liability; injury means someone else has to do your job. Your duty is to return to functioning, to maintain your equipment, which included your body. But at a certain point, I couldn't walk anymore. I came to understand that symptoms were my body crying out for help. Your body is not a never-ending resource; you can't always do more.

"I learned that I had to find a quiet space inside my own head. Otherwise, you wear yourself out trying to find it externally – the right drug, the right medicine, the right exercise, the right distraction. If you can find that quiet space, then it's yours any time you want. You can reset as many times as it takes. Until I learned that, I would use alcohol. When I couldn't take the physical pain anymore, I'd have a couple of drinks – 'Uncle Jack' [Daniels] helped me. The alcohol altered my mental state so I could tolerate things that were otherwise too depressing, too lonely, too physically and emotionally painful. It let me not be me for the next couple of hours – to get out of my head, to shut down the churning. Eventually, I decided I wanted to get better, and alcohol wasn't the way to do it.

"I've grown a whole lot in listening to my body, knowing that its symptoms are trying to tell me something. What does it want right now, what are its defenses, what makes it get activated, what helps it calm down? It's my job to learn its vocabulary. It may not be something pleasant, not something I want, but it's better than having something suppressed. I know now that symptoms are a manifestation of exceeding my coping ability – whether it's physical or mental. If you do too much of something, a symptom appears. You only get one body in this lifetime, so take care of it. Part of all this is radical acceptance. I had to face that I won't be able to do x, y, and z again. I used to try to get back to normal, but now I understand there's no back. You have to go forward to the new normal with the body you have starting today. It used to be 'Once I find the right doctor, I'm going to get back to work . . . once I find the right meds, once I find the right orthotics, once I find the right mattress, the right therapist, the right whatever – then I'll get back to normal.' But there's no back, ever. The world ends at your heels. All you have is what's in front of you."

18

Getting to a calm place:
The skill of *grounding*

No feeling is final.
—Rainer Maria Rilke, 20th-century German writer

All feelings are normal; they're part of being human. But if you have trauma or addiction, they can be too much or too little. Grounding helps you get them back to a healthy mid-level.

Most unsafe behavior occurs when you get stuck in strong negative feelings. If you can reduce them, you're less likely to act on them. Grounding is a lifeline back to shore, away from big waves of feeling.

Grounding means focusing outward on the external world – rather than inward toward the self. You can also think of it as *centering, calming, a safe place, looking outward, peacefulness,* or *healthy detachment*.

You can use grounding any time – before, during, or after a difficult situation. It works for *any* negative feeling: panic, anger, sadness, stress, fear, craving, triggering, dissociation, impulse to hurt someone, and so on. It uses simple but powerful strategies that you can do no matter where you are – on a bus, at work, in a classroom, while talking with someone, in line at the grocery store. Grounding is one of the most important recovery skills you can learn. "I wish I had learned it 20 years ago," said Marvin, a Vietnam veteran.

Three types of grounding are described in this chapter: *mental, physical,* and *soothing*. You can see which types work best for you. By rating your feelings before and after, you can also test how well grounding works.

In healthy families, children learn grounding informally by being comforted when in distress and by watching how others manage emotions. But if you didn't have the luck of growing up in a healthy family, you may not have learned how to shift out of negative feelings. You may find it hard to calm yourself. You may be so familiar with distress that it feels normal to you.

Many religious and spiritual traditions focus on healthy detachment. In "Trauma and Spirituality," Han van den Blink observes that detachment brings "freedom from the myriad thoughts, feelings, moods, ideologies, anxieties, worries, fears, and angers that continually pass through our minds and bodies and that so often hold us captive without our even being aware of it."

Healthy detachment doesn't mean being numb or not caring. It's being in touch with the present, centered and calm. Various methods such as meditation, mindfulness, and relaxation training can also bring forth such feelings. But those methods weren't designed to handle intense and dangerous impulses. Grounding is more active than those other approaches, and the eyes are kept open to keep you in touch with your environment. It was originally developed in psychiatric hospitals to help people, many with a history of trauma, regain a calmer state so that they wouldn't hurt themselves or others. If you're about to use a substance or punch a wall, for example, grounding can help.

See for yourself – try the following grounding exercises.

✶ Explore . . . *Try out grounding*

Guidelines

- Grounding can be done any time, anywhere, and no one has to know.

- Use grounding when you're faced with a trigger, having a flashback, dissociating, having a substance craving, or when your distress goes above 6 (on a 0–10 scale). Grounding puts healthy distance between you and these negative feelings.

- Keep your eyes open, scan the room, and turn the light on to stay in touch with the present.

- Rate your mood before and after to test whether it worked. Before grounding, rate your level of distress (0–10, where 10 means "intense distress"). Then rerate it afterward. Has it gone down?

- Stay neutral – no judgments of good and bad. For example, "The walls are blue; I dislike blue because it reminds me of depression." Simply say "The walls are blue" and move on.

- Focus on the present, not the past or future.

Step 1: Think of something moderately distressing – not the worst thing you can think of, but something that brings up some negative feelings. On a 0–10 scale, where 10 is the most intense distress, think of something between 5 and 7.

Step 2: Rate your level of distress from 0 (none) to 10 (intense distress). The goal will be to see if grounding helps to reduce the distress.

Step 3: Use as many of the following strategies as you can, in any order, until you reach 10 minutes total. And just do them; don't add in comments or judgments of good or bad.

EXAMPLES OF *MENTAL GROUNDING*

- *Describe your environment in detail* using all your senses. For example, "The walls are white, there are five pink chairs, there's a wooden bookshelf against the wall. . . . " Describe objects, sounds, textures, colors, smells, shapes, numbers, and temperature.

- *Play a categories game* with yourself. Try to think of "types of dogs," "jazz musicians," "states that begin with *A*," "cars," "TV shows," "writers," "sports," "songs," "cities."

- *Describe an everyday activity in great detail*. For example, describe a meal that you cook (e.g., "First I peel the potatoes, then I boil the water . . . ").

- *Imagine.* Use an image: glide along on skates away from your pain; change the TV channel to get to a better show.

- *Make a safety statement.* "My name is _____; I am safe right now. I am in the present, not the past. I am located in _____; the date is _____."

- *Use humor.* Think of something funny to jolt yourself out of your mood. Or read or watch some comedy.

EXAMPLES OF *PHYSICAL GROUNDING*

- *Run cool or warm water over your hands.*

- *Grab tightly on to your chair and notice what it feels like.*

- *Touch various objects around you*: a pen, keys, your clothing, the table, the walls. Notice textures, colors, materials, weight, temperature. Compare objects you touch. Is one colder? Lighter?

- *Dig your heels into the floor* – literally "grounding" them! Notice the tension centered in your heels as you do this. Remind yourself that you're connected to the ground.

- *Carry a grounding object in your pocket* – a small object (a small rock, clay, ring, piece of cloth or yarn) that you can touch whenever you feel triggered.
- *Jump up and down.*

EXAMPLES OF *SOOTHING GROUNDING*

- *Speak kindly to yourself* as if talking to a small child: "You're a good person going through a hard time. You'll get through this."
- *Think of favorites*: favorite color, animal, season, food, time of day, TV show, person, movie, activity, place, quotation, song, and scent. Also add other favorites you can think of.
- *Picture people you care about,* such as your children, and look at photographs of them.
- *Remember the words to an inspiring song, quotation, or poem* that makes you feel better, such as the Serenity Prayer.
- *Remember a safe place.* Describe a place that you find soothing (perhaps the beach or mountains or a favorite room).
- *Create a coping statement.* "I can handle it." "This feeling will pass."
- *Think of what you're looking forward to in the next week,* perhaps time with a friend or going to a movie.

Step 4: Afterward, rerate your negative feelings on the same scale from 0 (no distress) to 10 (intense distress). Did the number go down even a little? Do you feel even just a bit better than when you started? If not, try grounding again for 10 minutes. Then rerate your negative feelings again. If you try it long enough with enough different methods, it will work. See the next section for ideas.

*How to Boost Your Grounding**

Grounding works! But like any other skill, you need to practice to make it as powerful as possible. Below are suggestions to help make it work for you.

- **Practice as often as possible,** even when you don't need it, so that you'll know it by heart. Try it in different situations – when someone cuts you off in traffic; when you're stressed or depressed; or when you can't sleep at night.

---

*This list was adapted from *Seeking Safety* by Lisa M. Najavits (2002) with permission of the author.

- ***Practice faster.*** Speeding up the pace gets you focused on the outside world quickly.

- ***Try grounding for a loooooooonnnnnngggg time (20–30 minutes).*** And repeat, repeat, repeat.

- ***Try to notice which methods you like best*** – physical, mental, or soothing grounding methods, or some combination.

- ***Create your own methods of grounding.*** Any method you make up may be worth much more than those you read here, because it is *yours*.

- ***Start grounding early in a negative mood cycle:*** When a craving or flash-back is building, when anger is rising.

- ***Make a list*** of your best grounding methods and how long to use them.

- ***Have others assist you in grounding.*** Teach friends or family about ground-ing, so that they can help guide you with it if you become overwhelmed.

- ***Prepare in advance.*** Locate places at home, in your car, and at work where you have materials and reminders for grounding.

- ***Create a recording of a grounding message*** that you can play when needed. Consider asking your therapist or someone close to you to record it if you want to hear someone else's voice.

- ***Think about why grounding works.*** Why might it be that by focusing on the external world, you become more aware of an inner peacefulness? Notice the methods that work for you – why might those be more powerful for you than other methods?

- ***Don't give up!***

Grounding can become a positive emotional reflex, like "muscle memory," so that you have it when you need it.

◇ How does your body feel when you're grounded and calm?

◇ Which grounding methods work best for you?

◇ How can you remember to use grounding?

◇ In what situations do you most need to do grounding?

RECOVERY VOICES

Rita – "The first tool that helped me cope"

Rita served in the Army. "I learned not to feel. That's part of the mental tough-ness you learn in training that makes a soldier strong. I was at the top of my class and was respected by the guys (it was mostly guys there) because I could do what they did. I ran with the best of them. And I held my own at the bar. Drinking was part of Army life where I was stationed. Whenever something really good or really bad happened or when we were bored, we drank. So that was pretty much most nights. But it didn't get out of control for me until I was sexually assaulted by a soldier in my unit. After that, the drinking became a way to shut down the rage. I was afraid to report the attack because I had been drinking at the time and knew I'd be blamed. I tried to keep going, but inside I was falling apart. I drank more and more until I ended up getting arrested for driving drunk and hitting a parked car. I felt so ashamed. I had to go to a military hospital for psychiatric care, and that was the first time I started to see how the trauma had triggered serious drinking. I wish I knew then what I know now – that the alcohol kept me numb. I was on autopilot, trying to get through by pushing down feelings that tried to surface. I can see now that it doesn't work, but at the time it was all I knew. *Grounding* from Seeking Safety was the first tool that helped me cope because it's not about turning inward and trying to focus. My 'inward' was a mess, a scary place. Focusing on something concrete outside myself offered me a sense of con-trol the assault robbed me of 10 years ago."

19

The culture of silence

You didn't experience it, it never happened, you don't know what you know.

—From *Achilles in Vietnam: Combat Trauma and the Undoing of Character* (1994)

If I had known that my uncle had no right to touch me and that I could tell on him, then I might have yelled or screamed that night. If I'd known how we as a people are still struggling with the crippling effects of slavery and racism, I would have understood that my family silence after the secret came out was nothing personal. It was inspired by years of fear and oppression and passed on from one generation to the next.

—ROBIN STONE, *No Secrets No Lies: How Black Families Can Heal from Sexual Abuse* (2007)

More than many other issues, trauma and addiction are often met with silence. In response to addiction, families often create the fiction that everything is fine even when it's falling apart. With trauma, there may be intentional silencing (threatening a victim not to tell) or simply blindness to what's happening. People may say that your problems aren't all that bad or that it's better to put them out of mind. Pervasive silencing about trauma and addiction has also occurred in major institutions such as sports teams, the church, universities, corporations, and the military.

When no one acknowledges what's happening, you can doubt your reality. It feels crazy-making because we rely on others to help sort out our perceptions. It's been called "gaslighting" from the classic movie *Gaslight,* in which a woman gradually goes insane when her perceptions are repeatedly denied.

The phrase *culture of silence* conveys how strong a force silencing can be. People may say, "Why didn't you speak up?" or "You should have told someone," not under-standing how culture – in a family, community, or institution – can create extraor-dinary pressure *not* to speak up. Breaking the silence is often dangerous. There's an implied or sometimes direct threat that you will be rejected, humiliated, put down, or physically harmed. And the more extreme the problem, the more extreme the silenc-ing becomes. As with the famous monkeys, "see no evil, hear no evil, speak no evil" becomes a way for serious problems to flourish.

Silence also leads to terrible isolation that can add to the pain of trauma and addiction. If you were isolated after trauma, you may have felt misunderstood, may have doubted your memories, and may never have received support. Silencing is one of the primary ways that trauma perpetrators are able to get away with what they do. They instill in the victim an inability to talk about trauma by creating threats ("If you talk about it, I will _____") or invalidating the victim's experience by making trauma seem normal. In cases of neglect, there may be the message that "You want and need too much; you're the problem, not me."

Some trauma survivors feel guilty that they didn't speak up. But silence likely reflected deep knowledge. You knew what was expected, and staying quiet may have saved you from worse harm. You may also have dissociated or denied to yourself how awful it was, which are automatic self-protection mechanisms in which your mind shuts down when there's too much pain. These innate instincts for survival represent the escape when there's no escape, "one of nature's small mercies" in the words of Judith Herman in *Trauma and Recovery*.

It can take years for some trauma victims to reclaim their story, rebuilding it piece by piece as part of counseling, validation by other survivors, and other healing methods. People who go through trauma as part of a community, such as a hurricane or terrorist incident, often have quicker recovery because there is a shared reality with others.

Addiction, too, has silencing. It often goes unseen, unspoken. You learn not to bring it up because no one speaks of it as a problem. It becomes invisible and then totally acceptable.

Katrina describes the attitude toward drinking that she observed in the Army. "Drinking was all but encouraged. We had beer machines in the barracks. In the movies, you could drink. Even though there were rations for some stuff, you could get as much alcohol as you wanted. Video games were big too. It was like a frat. Why was alcohol so much a part of things? Partly it was because there was a lot of trauma – 'I can take a left turn down alcohol road and I'll keep stuff down that I don't want to see.' Also, there was boredom; there wasn't a lot else to do. And it wasn't seen as a problem. The attitude was 'I just medicate with alcohol, but I'm not an addict.' It was only a problem if you had clear and obvious consequences, like not showing up for duty or getting into a big fight or a DUI. I think it would help if they asked questions like 'Have you ever underreported your drinking and why? Do you think you should drink less? Are you disappointed by how much you drink? Would you feel better about yourself if you drank less?' Those might get people to see a problem sooner."

There are deep power dynamics that support cultures of silence. Paulo Freire, a 1970s Brazilian educator and philosopher, coined the term *culture of silence* based on his observations about oppressed people. Those without social power "are not heard by the dominant members of their society" and "internalize negative images of themselves." Trauma and addiction are both rooted in powerlessness. When you feel that you don't have power, you become silent. Recovery is the opposite – coming into your truth, owning it, and, if you choose to, voicing it to safe people.

✧ Do you feel that you were not believed about your trauma? Your addiction?

✧ Do you have difficulty hanging on to your own truth?

✧ Do you flip back and forth in your view about your trauma? Your addiction?

✧ Do you feel that people have taken your trauma seriously? Your addiction?

Suggestions for Breaking the Silence

There is no one way to break silence. It may mean opening up to specific people about your experiences. It may mean journaling to explore your own truth. It may mean taking legal action if it's relevant to do that. Whatever you choose to do, consider the suggestions on pages 134–135.

Try small experiments. Open up in small ways until you see whether someone is trustworthy and able to support you. Gradually build trust and vulnerability in relationships.

Don't worry about looking stupid. It will feel awkward to bring up difficult topics. Stay focused on your goal.

Assess for safety. Always be careful to evaluate whether there's potential danger for you, either physical or emotional. Get input from as many safe people as possible, such as counselors and friends. If you don't know whether anyone can be trusted, work on the "small experiments" described above.

Be patient with yourself. Overcoming silence can take a long time, so be patient as you work on it. You may instinctively stay quiet even in situations where it now may be safe to speak up. Your reactions may be so automatic that you don't even notice them.

Understand that much of the work is internal. In silencing you become unknown even to yourself. You may wonder: "Does my trauma really matter?" "Maybe it wasn't so bad?" "Do I really have an addiction?" It's common to flip back and forth between extremes: "I'm fine/I'm a mess"; "It was awful/It wasn't that bad"; "I can recover/It's hopeless." As you recover, you'll find greater wholeness – the ability to sustain a consistent view of yourself.

Never voice serious issues when intoxicated. In the moment, it may feel right to say things you'll later regret. So no "drunk texting" or discussion of major issues while you're intoxicated.

Don't confront a trauma perpetrator if you're in early recovery. You may have an apology fantasy – that if you confront someone who harmed you, you'll get the apology you've always wanted. But you may be deeply disappointed. Many trauma survivors find that not only do they not get the apology but confrontation may evoke emotional and even physical harm. Families often rally around the perpetrator rather than the victim. Confronting a trauma perpetrator is very challenging and should not be done when you're in early recovery from trauma or addiction. Focus on yourself for now. The only exception is if you have to testify for legal proceedings, which needs to be done with a lawyer's guidance.

Plan, don't be impulsive, when speaking your truth. It's common when overcoming years of silence to move too quickly from silence to speech. You may start "spilling" inappropriately to people who may not be able to hear it. Other than in counseling, where you can express yourself freely, prepare how you'll speak to others so that it'll have the best chance of success. Be clear on your goals and what you want to say and run it by people you trust.

Learn more about breaking silence. Search online. There are also various books on how to bring up difficult topics.

> ✧ Are there silences that you want to break? Is it safe to do so? How might you go about it?

RECOVERY VOICES

Becky – "Just talking about silencing makes the silence less powerful."

"Not only did my family deny my trauma (I was molested by my brother-in-law from ages 8 to 10), but they told me that I should stop talking nonsense about our family. So I came to the conclusion that it must be me. My mother took me to the doctor to get me a prescription and he gave me Valium. I thought there must be something wrong with me, but what? What was so terribly wrong with me that even my own family can't speak about what happened to me? What was so attractive about an 8-year-old child that caused a grown man to hurt me like that? What caused my family to believe that we shouldn't talk about any of this? I took a drink, the drink took a drink, and on it went, feeding my addiction. My brother-in-law died many years later, and my mother's last words to me about this were, 'We do not speak ill of the dead.' So now he's still keeping me silent because he's dead? When I was a child I prayed for the abuse to stop, and later he died. Something in me said it must be me that killed him by praying for that, even though I knew it wasn't true. And still to this day, 45 years later, I have not talked about it with my family. I've been in successful recovery from trauma and alcohol abuse for decades now, and here's what I've learned about silencing. It's hard work to break the silence, but 'If it's mentionable, then it's manageable,' as Mr. Rogers, the children's TV show host, famously said. I was able to open up to people outside my family – not a lot of people, but enough to help me heal. Just talking about silencing makes the silence less powerful, and secrets can be spoken of more and more. Listening is also an important vehicle for healing – repair happens by hearing people who have suffered in ways that seem a little like your own. It's been a hard road but well worth the journey."

20

Motivation: Leverage one problem
to help another

Not knowing when the dawn will come I open every door.
—EMILY DICKINSON, 19th-century American poet

It can be hard to find the will to turn your life around. You may feel worn out, hopeless.

Michele was 13 when she survived a very rare medication allergy that brought on toxic epidermal necrolysis syndrome, destroying her entire outer layer of skin like a full-body burn patient. She recovered physically but developed PTSD that lasted for years. She writes, "The beginning of my recovery looked like this:

1. Force me to go to therapy for one hour, once a week.

2. I show up and expect the therapist to do all of the work.

3. For the rest of the week, I pretend there's nothing else to do and just try to limp through the days coping with symptoms.

Why did I pretend there was nothing else to do? Because if you've ever, for a second, struggled with the effects of trauma or PTSD, you know what it feels like to be sleep deprived, depressed, emotionally volatile, powerless, hopeless, and sometimes just downright utterly despondent. In that state of mind, I often believed there was no way to save me. I was crazy and would remain so forever.

The effects of trauma on mind, body, and soul can cause enormous fatigue that saps any motivating energy source. Yet overcoming trauma and PTSD means you absolutely must find a way to feel motivated or compelled to take the necessary actions to move forward."

—From *Get Your Brain Motivated to Recover from PTSD*, by Michele Rosenthal

---

When you're stuck, motivation seems like something you either have or you don't. Like money, once it's gone it's gone. But motivation is a fluid asset – you can increase it by thinking about it in new ways. You can find the *how* if you create a *why*. Leveraging your motivation is a key way to do that.

Leverage One Problem Off Another

Leveraging one problem off another means you find something you're more motivated to work on and use that to inspire yourself to work on something you're less motivated to work on. It's a two-for-one strategy – "A rising tide lifts all boats," as the saying goes. Here are examples of what it might sound like.

> "*I want to be the best parent I can be.* It's hard to work on my PTSD, but unless I do that, my kids won't have a healthy, stable parent."

> "*I really want to find a life partner.* But unless I work on my sex addiction I'll find myself 10 years out with a trail of hookups and no real relationship."

In these examples, the first sentence describes something the person feels motivated to work on (being a good parent, finding a life partner). In the second sentence, the person links it to something he or she is not so motivated to work on (PTSD, sex addiction).

> ✧ Fill in the following sentence: "I really want to achieve _____. To do that, I need to work on _____, even if I don't feel like it."

Trauma and Addiction Motivation

If you have both addiction and trauma problems, you may feel more motivated to work on one than the other. This is common.

Usually, trauma is more motivating. No one chooses trauma, and no one wants the feelings that arise from it – flashbacks, nightmares, depression, anger, and so on. Addiction may be less clear: you're the one picking up the drug, the porn, or the credit card, and the addictive behavior feels good, at least for a while. Even once it's a problem you may be the last to see it, as it's typically more visible to people around you (family and friends, employers, doctors, or the police).

You can leverage whichever one – trauma or addiction – you have more motivation for. For example:

Trauma is the motivation: "I'm a survivor; I lived through awful trauma and want to heal from that. My counselor tells me that I have to work on my alcohol problems too. Maybe she's right that working on both will speed up my recovery."

Addiction is the motivation: "All along I thought my problem was just addiction, and I worked hard on that. But now I see my trauma problems were underneath, driving the addiction. I'll have to work on both."

In each example, the person is more motivated on one than the other but is open to the idea of working on both at the same time. That's the goal.

"Hijacked" Motivation

Motivation is a complex topic. In addiction and trauma, motivation can get directed toward unhealthy goals. This is called *hijacked* motivation – spending large amounts of time and energy in ways that reinforce addiction or trauma.

For example, after Lorna survived a rape her life became more and more narrow. She spent hours every day checking the locks on her doors and windows, going through each room to make sure no one was there, and creating barricades in case of an intruder. Her daily life became an obsessive routine that was defined by her trauma.

In short, you may have a lot of motivation, but it may be directed toward expressions of your illness rather than toward recovery. So the task is to direct your energy, your life force, toward what builds you up rather than keeps you down.

✵ Explore . . . *Your motivation*

The following questions can help you reflect on your motivations so as to create more leverage for recovery. There are no right or wrong answers. If you have just trauma problems (no addiction) or vice versa, skip questions that don't apply to you.

1. What life goal are you *most* motivated to work on right now? (For example: To be a better parent? Get a better job? Go back to school? Find a partner? Make more money? Move to a better neighborhood? Help others?)

_____

_____

   a. How can addiction recovery help you move toward that goal?

      _____

      _____

   b. How can trauma recovery help you move toward that goal?

      _____

      _____

2. From 0 to 10 (0 = not at all; 10 = greatly), how motivated are you to work on:

   a. Your trauma problems? _____

   b. Your addiction? _____

3. From 0 to 10 (0 = not at all; 10 = greatly), how much does your motivation feel "hijacked" toward unhealthy goals in relation to:

   a. Your trauma problems? _____

   b. Your addictions? _____

4. If one area improves, might it help the other too?

   a. If your addiction improves, how might that help your trauma recovery?

      _____

      _____

   b. If your trauma problems improve, how might that help your addiction recovery?

      _____

      _____

5. Are there any inspiring words, quotes, examples, or ideas that increase your motivation to work on your:

   a. Trauma recovery?

      _____

      _____

   b. Addiction recovery?

      _____

      _____

RECOVERY VOICES

Travis – "A chance at something better"

"I'm a firefighter and have seen a lot of bad stuff. I think I've had PTSD for years, but till recently I felt like I would've rather died than talk to anyone about it. Where I work, physical accomplishment is praised and emotional weakness is ridiculed. I also didn't want to get help because I was using a fair amount of cocaine and knew it might cost me my job due to zero-tolerance policies. So I shut up and put up. One of the ways I avoided dealing with stuff was to throw myself into something physical, working out too hard and signing up for too many shifts. It's an adrenaline rush. The end result is that I'm exhausted, worn out in body and spirit. The section in this chapter called 'hijacked motivation' really speaks to me. I've been motivated toward a lot of destructive behavior – not just the too-intense physical stuff but also fits of anger, which have physically and emotionally damaged some people, including my girlfriend. I get it now that motivation isn't always positive. You have to be motivated toward the right things that will bring good that lasts. I'm early in recovery from PTSD and not sure I can make it. Sometimes I think it's better not to try at all if I might fail. But I know that if I keep going on the same old path I'll either burn up or burn out. I can't keep doing what I've been doing. I guess you could call this motivation. At least it's a starting place that gives me a chance at something better."

21

Tip the Scales recovery plan

> . . . always remember: You are braver than you believe, stronger
> than you seem, and smarter than you think.
> —A. A. MILNE, 20th-century British author of *Winnie-the-Pooh*

The bottom line of recovery is to *increase your safe behavior and decrease your unsafe behavior.*

Behaviors that you're trying to decrease may be addiction related (excessive drinking, drugging, spending, eating, gambling, etc.); trauma related (isolation, harming yourself or other people, etc.); or a mix.

The goal is to tip the scales in a healthy direction. It's like a seesaw where you increase the weight on the safe behaviors side and decrease the weight on the unsafe behaviors side.

By focusing on what you're *adding in* (safe behavior) as well as *taking out* (unsafe behavior) you'll be better able to manage one of the big fears in early recovery – that you can't live without the unsafe behavior. For some people, letting go of the unsafe behavior is like facing a dark abyss, an empty pit, and they believe they'll just be stuck in horrible feelings that they won't be able to tolerate. But the reality is much more dynamic, interesting, and optimistic. It's a growth process of building yourself up with lots of help along the way. We're using the term *tip the scales* because you don't have to do it perfectly; rather, it's about aiming in the right direction as much as you can.

In this chapter, there are six questions to answer that can help you create your Tip the Scales plan. Go ahead and create the plan even if it seems like it can't work or you've tried things like this before. Putting a plan on paper and trying it out is simple but profound. Research shows that plans like this help improve mood and functioning even if you don't believe they'll work.

If you're not clear what your safe and unsafe behaviors are, see "Listen to your behavior" (Chapter 7). That chapter also has alternate language if you don't like the terms *safe* and *unsafe*.

☆ Explore . . . *Create your Tip the Scales recovery plan*

This exercise is a series of questions; just go one by one.

Step 1: *Decrease an Unsafe Behavior*

Answer the following three questions and read the information below each question for guidance to help your plan succeed.

(a) **What is the unsafe behavior you want to *decrease?*** _____

Examples: ▪ "Drinking too much" ▪ "Yelling at my partner" ▪ "Bingeing on junk food" ▪ "Hanging with violent people" ▪ "Excessive gaming" ▪ "Overeating" ▪ "Watching too much porn" ▪ "Cutting" ▪ "Time on the Internet" ▪ "Isolating" ▪ "Drugging" ▪ "Too much TV"

For now, focus on just one key unsafe behavior; you can work on others later. Choose a behavior that's currently damaging to you or others in your life – one that really needs to change. If needed, see "Listen to your behavior" (Chapter 7) to identify a behavior to work on.

(b) **How much are you currently* doing the unsafe behavior per week?** _____

Examples: ▪ "I drink a bottle of wine a day" ▪ "I spend about $300 on gambling a week" ▪ "I binge on food three times a week" ▪ "I cut myself twice a week on average" ▪ "I take seven pain pills a day when I party, which is about three nights a week, so that's 21 pills a week" ▪ "I eat sweets six times a day, so that's about 42 times a week (6 × 7 days)" ▪ "I yell at my partner about three times a day, so that's about 21 times a week (3 × 7 days)"

Your answer will depend on the type of behavior. It could be *number of dollars, bottles, pills,* or *times per week*, for example. Be specific and focus on what's typical for you, even if it varies from week to week.

Take a moment to really think about this question. Many people aren't aware how often they're doing an unsafe behavior; they just know it's too much. This

---

*"Currently" means the most typical week in the past month.

question may feel uncomfortable, as the unsafe behavior may be happening a lot more than you think. Whatever the truth is, you can work to make it better.

(c) **What's your target goal for your unsafe behavior?**

"I want to decrease my _____ behavior to _____."

Examples:

"I want to decrease my <u>TV watching</u> behavior to <u>1 hour per day</u>."

"I want to decrease my <u>cutting</u> behavior to <u>0 times per day</u>."

"I want to decrease my <u>cocaine use</u> behavior to <u>0 times per day</u>."

"I want to decrease my <u>drinking</u> behavior to <u>1 ounce hard liquor 3 times per week</u>."

"I want to decrease my <u>gambling</u> behavior to <u>2 times, $25 each time ($50 total), per month</u>.

Three Types of Recovery Goals

As you identify your target, choose what's healthiest for you among the choices below.

ABSTINENCE

In this approach, you commit to giving up the behavior entirely. It applies to behavior where this is possible, such as substances, self-harm behavior, and gambling, rather than work, food, or spending, which you have to do to survive. Abstinence is always the best way to go if you're willing to do it. It's also essential if you have a serious problem with the behavior or it's gone on for a long time.

If you're choosing abstinence, your answer would be "0" per day to question (c) above. For example, "I want to decrease my <u>cutting</u> behavior to <u>0 times per day</u>."

HARM REDUCTION

This approach means that you gradually decrease the unsafe behavior rather than giving it up totally right now. If you're smoking weed every day, for example, you could set a goal of smoking every other day. It's called *harm reduction,* as the idea is to start reducing the harm in whatever way is possible for you – "Fifty percent of something is better than 100% of nothing." This approach is typically used for people who aren't willing to commit to abstinence right now. Harm reduction is often used as a path toward later abstinence.

If you're choosing harm reduction, list your limit for question (c). For example, "I want to decrease my <u>drinking</u> behavior to <u>1 ounce hard liquor per day.</u>"

CONTROLLED USE

Controlled use is the idea that people who have only a *mild problem* may be able to return to safe levels of the behavior. Controlled use may be worth trying if you're catching the problem early, you're highly motivated to succeed, you're doing well in other parts of your life, and your problem is definitely mild. See "It's medical – you're not crazy, lazy, or bad" (Chapter 4) for how *mild* is defined. If your problem is serious or long-standing, abstinence (or harm reduction followed by abstinence) is strongly recommended and likely to be the only healthy option for you.

Even if you believe you may be able to succeed at controlled use, it's strongly advised to start with at least 30 days of no use at all and then try controlled use. This promotes success by allowing you to create a new habit from scratch. Also, if you can't do 30 days without any use, you likely have a serious addiction, in which case controlled use would not be healthy for you.

If you're choosing controlled use, list your limit for the question (c) on the previous page. For example, "For the next month I won't gamble at all. After that, I'll <u>gamble</u> no more than <u>two times, $25 each time ($50 total) per month.</u>"

Whatever your goal, make it specific. It doesn't work to just say, "I'll try to cut down." You really may believe you can do it less, but you'll likely end up doing it more than you intend. So be clear on your goal: how much and how often. This way, you can measure your success each week. For the time frame, choose what's best for you. Some commit to a day at a time; others to a week, a month, or sometimes their entire lifetime.

Step 2: *Increase Safe Behavior*

Now answer the two questions on the next page. To create lasting change, it's just as important to *increase your safe behavior* as it is to *decrease your unsafe behavior.*

Wherever you direct your attention, your energy follows. Picture pulling the reins on a horse to steer it in a new direction. Your energy is currently directed toward your unsafe behavior, so the idea is to turn and steer away from that.

Safe behaviors buy you time to "rewire" your brain so that, over time, unsafe behavior won't feel so powerful. At first you'll still have urges toward the unsafe behavior, but those will go down over time. Everyone can create new habits. Many people with even the most severe unsafe behavior have built successful recovery. Even if you don't believe it'll happen for you, just keep going with this plan.

(a) **What safe behaviors do you want to *increase?* (circle them below)**

Stay active and just keep doing anything at all – as long as it's safe – to build your recovery "muscles." Choose activities you find fun, useful, or that just fill time. Take up your mental space with distractions from cravings.

Circle as many as you can that are realistic and healthy for you.

Examples: ▪ Call a safe friend or family member ▪ Try on different clothing or hairstyles ▪ Take a shower ▪ Paint your room ▪ Help someone who needs help ▪ Go to the library ▪ Cook a meal ▪ Take your dog for a walk ▪ Sort laundry ▪ Organize friends to go on an outing ▪ Go bowling ▪ Go to the gym ▪ Start learning something new ▪ Go to a self-help meeting ▪ Get some rest ▪ Enter a treatment program ▪ Do *grounding* ▪ Clean a room ▪ Get work done ▪ Browse in a store ▪ Answer emails ▪ Listen to an audiobook or music ▪ Go to your church or other religious place ▪ Look for a course to take online or at a local school ▪ Go outside and take some interesting photos and then write captions for them ▪ Call a hotline ▪ Sort through some clutter ▪ Do a safe hobby ▪ Paint, draw, or write ▪ Watch TV or a movie ▪ Go for a run ▪ Look into volunteering ▪ Attend an electronic (phone) self-help meeting ▪ Fix something at home that needs fixing (but not another person!) ▪ Shop for food ▪ Read recovery information online ▪ Ask others to tell you about their recovery process ▪ Create a calendar to keep track of your schedule ▪ Play with your kids ▪ Read the news ▪ Write fun lists (favorite things, your strengths, places you want to visit, etc.) ▪ Play a game ▪ Go to a concert ▪ Pray ▪ Build something (a carpentry project) ▪ Bike ▪ Meditate ▪ Try a new recipe

Others?

_____

_____

_____

Keep going until you have as long a list as possible.

(b) i. **How many hours per day do you *currently spend on* safe behaviors?** _____

   ii. **How many hours per day do you *want to spend on* safe behaviors?** _____

Whatever your current number of hours of safe behavior, increase them. It's a simple but powerful calculation: the more hours you devote to safe behaviors, the stronger your recovery. It's a numbers game – soak up your time and energy with more and more. It gets you away from the chatter in your head that draws you back to unsafe behavior. It's like changing the TV to a new channel.

Step 3: *Track Your Safe and Unsafe Behaviors*

Keep track of your safe and unsafe behaviors for a while. Try it for a week and see how it feels. It doesn't have to be perfect and doesn't have to become a big job. Small efforts pay big rewards. You'll be able to see even subtle changes that aren't visible otherwise. This sets off a positive feedback loop; you can take pride in tipping the scales in the right direction. If the tracking shows a worsening problem, you'll be more aware of it early on so you can figure out what to do about it. Either way you win – you maintain forward progress. Awareness is an important friend in recovery. Like a good friend, it's honest with you to help you grow.

Here are some ways to keep track.

- *Electronic methods.* Search for "daily diary" online and you'll find free tools to track behaviors you choose. You can set up text or email prompts and store the tracking on your phone or tablet.

- *Use a timer.* This can be a very satisfying method. You set a kitchen timer or phone timer and stick with the safe behavior for a defined period, such as a half hour, hour, or 2 hours. When the timer goes off, you decide what your next safe behavior will be and set the timer again.

- *Use a printed calendar.* Use a simple hard-copy daily diary. Fill it in ongoing (best way) or at the end of the day.

Success Strategies

Boost your plan with the following methods. The more you do, the more you'll tip the scales toward recovery.

◇ Circle at least five methods to try.

○ *Create a why and it will lead you to how.* Do it because you've suffered enough. Do it because your kids will get their mom or dad back.

○ *Make it fun.* Be playful: fill a small container with pieces of paper, each with a safe behavior on it. Pull one out at random and do it, then pull another and do that, and so on. You can create an electronic version of this game using a free online random picker (search that phrase online to find one). Or just write out a list of safe behaviors, and when it's time to pick one close your eyes, point anywhere on the list, open your eyes, and go do that one. Keep the list in your wallet or on your phone so you can use it whenever you need to get away from unsafe behavior.

○ *Watch for the all-or-none trap.* In addiction, it's called the *abstinence violation effect*: if you have a slip you think, "I failed my plan, so I might as well keep drinking." To counteract this, try to view it as a continuous line rather than an all-or-none switch. It's like a ski slope – learn to slow down and stop rather than sliding all the way downhill into relapse.

○ *Share it with people who want you to succeed.* The more you share your plan, the more likely you are to stick with it. Choose people who want you to succeed. Some people may feel threatened or try to undermine you if they see you moving forward.

○ *How long? At least a half hour at a time.* That's the time it takes to decrease most cravings and urges. Keep stacking half hour on half hour. Keep tipping the scale.

○ *Remember "progress, not perfection."* Many people with addiction and trauma problems spiral into self-loathing when they fall short. Keep trying, and when you make a mistake jump back in and try again.

○ *Know what to expect.* Early on, you'll likely have cravings and inner conflict (the "angel/devil" on your shoulder). You may also feel easily triggered – a sunset reminds you of drinking; a computer reminds you of porn. Know that it'll definitely get easier if you stick with your plan. Listen to anyone who's done successful recovery to hear what it's like. Eventually the cravings, inner conflict, and triggers really do subside.

○ *Consider entering a treatment program.* If you've been using heavily or can't reduce your use even when trying your hardest, get into treatment. It could be counseling, self-help groups, a medication doctor, addiction rehab, or psychiatric care. Don't go it alone. For options, see "Listen to your behavior" (Chapter 7), "Find your way" (Chapter 9), or "Two types of trauma counseling" (Chapter 33).

○ *Give your plan a name.* Here I Am Plan, Tip the Scales Log, Recovery Calendar, or any other.

○ *Remove temptation.* Protect yourself from triggers. Your brain is like a dog leaping at a bone when it sees reminders of your unsafe behavior such as a liquor store or a casino. As they say in AA, "Change people, places, and things." Take a different route to work to avoid the liquor store; file a form with a casino to voluntarily block yourself from being allowed in (called *self-exclusion*). Create obstacles to your triggers.

o **Keep it visible.** Use any methods that keep your plan front and center. Keep a copy in your wallet so you see it when you reach for money; put it on your phone; create a daily reminder in your calendar; give a copy to someone who cares about you and review it together each week.

o **For now, ignore your feelings.** You may say, "It's too hard," "I'm too depressed to do this," or "I'm numb and don't care anymore." The Tip the Scales plan is not about feelings. It's a simple, elegant plan: replace unsafe behavior with safe behavior over and over until you feel it in your bones and make it pure instinct. You may love it, hate it, be neutral toward it, fear it, feel down about it. You can have any feelings at all, but stick with it.

o **Reward yourself.** For each day or week you stick to your plan, give yourself a healthy reward. If you don't meet your target, identify what you can improve and try again tomorrow, this time with some new coping.

o **Do something, anything.** Just keep doing *anything* that's safe for you. Take a walk or drive if you can't think of anything else. Listen to music. Cook a meal. It's just simple things again and again.

o **Don't be seduced by "maybe."** Maybe usually means no. So no *no*'s or *maybe*s. Just *yes*.

o **Give it 30 days.** Studies show it takes 30 days to create a new habit. Stick with it.

o **Use all the coping skills you can.** See "Safe coping skills" (Chapter 12) and "Getting to a calm place: The skill of grounding" (Chapter 18) and any other chapters that offer ideas for dealing with challenges.

o **Now – not later.** You may be tempted to say, "I'll quit tomorrow" or "Just one more." Start right now and keep working on it every chance you get. Replace your unsafe behavior with safe behavior, over and over and over.

✧ Can you promise yourself you'll try the plan for at least a week?

✧ Who can you share your plan with so they can help you stick with it?

RECOVERY VOICES

David – "My actions never lie."

"I really appreciate this chapter; it helps me pay attention. My behavior is the best barometer of how I am doing. My head is sometimes like this big fog-shrouded landscape. I feel like I can't see where I'm going and there's potential danger right in front of me but I can't see it. By tracking my actions as safe and unsafe, I begin to have a sort of map of where I am and how I'm doing. The thing about addiction and PTSD is they are full of lies so I can never really trust my thinking. The Tip the Scales plan is an effective tool for me to start heading in the right direction. The plan makes sense. If I use drugs, engage in a porn binge, cut myself, or binge and purge, and keep track of when and how much I do that, after a short time I can see patterns of when I am most in distress, and maybe I find by keeping track I am in more distress than I realize. It's easy to lose track of time when getting high and sometimes dissociating. Keeping track of all my behaviors, like how much money I'm spending on drugs, meals, porn, shopping, is immensely helpful. I'm the one keeping track, so the facts are from me. It's hard to argue against myself, although I might try. Tracking positive activities is also helpful. I can see connections between not getting rest, skipping meals, and negative behaviors. I also like that the chapter talks about not judging myself about the behaviors and not putting pressure on myself to change everything at once. Before I can change I need to know exactly what needs changing and where I need to start. The most helpful aspect of this chapter for me is that it helps me determine exactly where I am, not where I think I am. I think of scuba diving. When underwater, a diver can very easily lose a sense of which way is up. Were that diver to swim downward instead of toward the surface, he could be facing death. But his air bubbles guide him to the surface – they never lie. My behaviors tell me exactly how I'm doing, so this chapter is helpful and a logical approach. I might not always tell the truth, but my actions never lie."

22

Every child is a detective

Every family is a mystery; every child is a detective.
—SHARON O'BRIEN, American writer

Family history is one of the biggest predictors of both addiction and trauma problems. If you have relatives with addiction, you're more likely to have addiction; and so, too, if your family has trauma problems you're more likely to have trauma problems. It's called *intergenerational* trauma and addiction: both tend to carry across generations unless recovery becomes a priority.

You can break the cycle. It's not an automatic life script. Most children of alcoholics don't develop substance problems, for example (about 36% do); and most people abused as children don't go on to abuse their own children (about 30% do).

One way to help break the cycle is to become aware of the messages you absorbed growing up. You live what you learned, yet you learned it mostly unaware, unstated. It was just part of growing up.

Messages that play a role in addiction include:

» "Live for today."
» "Your money is your worth."
» "Food is love."
» "Alcohol is the way to relax."

Messages that play a role in trauma include:

» "Pretend things are fine."
» "Violence is normal."
» "Don't feel."
» "Your needs don't matter."

Such messages create a powerful force field in your life. The quote at the start of this chapter captures the idea: "Every family is a mystery; every child is a detective." Children figure out the rules of their family. They have to in order to survive.

The goal now is to look at the broad context beyond you as an individual – to explore messages you absorbed that help explain the development and persistence of your addiction and trauma problems. You're the product of many influences, including your family, peers, ethnicity, gender, generation, media, institutions (such as schools, religious institutions, the military), jobs you hold, political beliefs you're exposed to, your physical environment, music you listen to, and many others. You may be aware of only some of these. Usually, the strongest influences are those you're not aware of. It's said that culture is unconscious. Some cultures value personal expression; others value conformity. Some value a strict power structure; others value equality. Some promote addictive behavior; others discourage it. There are many cultural messages you can absorb.

> ✧ Identify one major *helpful* message you absorbed from your family or community and one *unhelpful* message you absorbed.

Early social messages become part of who you are. They are building blocks of consciousness. They show up in the choices you make, what you value, what you tolerate, who you like and dislike, how you communicate, and much else. They can shift over time, and you may want to keep some but reject others. Some may have a positive influence on you, some negative, and some neutral. Messages can become unhealthy when they're rigid or extreme. They don't allow you to adapt to different situations. Flexibility is part of healthy survival.

Keep in mind, too, that the same message may have a different impact depending on who delivers it and how it's delivered. The message "food is love" can build warm family bonds around the dinner table or can lead to an eating disorder. Notice the messages you absorbed and how they affect you.

✮ Explore . . . *Choose the messages you want to keep*

Which messages do you want to keep? Which will help you create the life you want?

On pages 152–153, the left column lists messages that are largely *unhealthy* and the right column lists messages that are usually *healthy* – but remember that it depends on the context, so read them carefully. There are no right or wrong answers. It's about becoming aware.

Step 1: The messages *you learned as a child*

Circle those in each column *that you grew up with*. These are ones you didn't get to choose; they were part of your environment. They may likely include a mix of both healthy and unhealthy messages.

Step 2: The messages *you want to live by as an adult*

Next, go through the table and put a star next to *those you want to live by* now. No matter what you grew up with, you can choose the messages you want to keep going forward.

Messages

Unhealthy	Healthy
Don't trust.	Good people can be trusted.
Food is love.	Food is food.
Stuff your feelings.	Value your feelings.
If you can't say something nice, don't say anything.	Anything can be talked about if said kindly.
You won't amount to anything.	You can go far.
Substances solve problems.	Substances aren't a real solution.
Don't make waves.	Strive for what you want.
Your worth is your work.	You have value beyond your achievements.
Take what is given to you.	Ask for what you want.
It's okay to give up.	Never give up.
Life should be easy.	Life is a struggle; you have to work at it.

Messages

Unhealthy	Healthy
You're less important than others.	You're as important as others.
Look out for yourself.	We're all in it together.
Children should be seen and not heard.	Children can express themselves.
Conflicts can't be talked about.	Conflicts can be aired and resolved.
Other people have it all together.	Everyone struggles.
Your money and possessions show what you're worth.	You're worthwhile regardless of money and possessions.
It's threatening to others if you achieve more than they do.	Rise as high as you can.
Addiction is your own fault.	Addiction is a medical illness.
You brought trauma on yourself.	No one chooses trauma.
Life is just stress.	Life includes joy.
Might makes right.	Integrity matters.
Appearance is everything.	Who you are is everything.

Any other *healthy* messages you absorbed from your family? _____

_____

Any other *unhealthy* messages you absorbed? _____

_____

Reflections . . .

Take a broad view. Explore your many early influences – people, media, communities, culture, and family history.

No shame, no blame. Notice, with an open heart, what influenced you so that you can feel more compassion for how you ended up where you are now. No judgments – just insight.

Remember there are many reasons for trauma and addiction problems. This chapter explores just one aspect: early social messages.

RECOVERY VOICES

Jade – "The messages were so embedded in our family story."

"I was neglected growing up, so I learned most things by their absence rather than their presence. This chapter helps me see that I was absorbing messages all along, even though no one sat down and said them out loud. Because I had so little interaction with the 'very successful' adults in my life, I didn't learn that life was a continual effort. I took to drugs as soon as I had access to them in middle school because I really believed I was supposed to feel good all the time and didn't know how to do that on my own. The drugs helped until, of course, they didn't.

"I grew up in a wealthy home, but my parents were functioning alcoholics. I learned some of the lessons so well that it's hard for me to change them, even though they aren't all that useful. The biggest of those was 'don't trust.' What I saw was all about keeping up appearances but never being vulnerable inside or outside the family. It was like a game or a theater piece, and the idea was to play it well. I never knew what to do with what I now know were regular childhood feelings: fear, confusion, shame, awkwardness. Some other messages help and hurt me at the same time, so it's a challenge when deciding how much I should let them go. For example, 'You are your achievements,' and 'Conflicts are to be avoided.' These helped me succeed in my work but stunted my relationships.

"The opening quote to this chapter sums up how I feel. In fact, the messages were so embedded in our family story that it took me until my early midlife to uncover their mystery."

23

How to survive a relapse

Fail again. Fail better.
—SAMUEL BECKETT, 20th-century Irish playwright and winner
of the Nobel Prize in Literature

To *relapse* means to backslide, to have a setback after a period of improvement. You succeeded in reducing a behavior for a while but then began doing it again. Relapse is most discussed in relation to addiction but can occur for any behavior you're trying to change – such as returning to a partner who hurt you, shame-filled secretive behaviors, or yelling at people.

The term *slip* is used for backsliding that is less severe or intense. You may have had one drink, for example, and then quickly got yourself back on track into abstinence. The following tips can help with both slips and relapses.

What to Do for an *Addiction* Relapse

Right after a relapse is a very vulnerable time. It's easy to turn against yourself and berate yourself, which is so discouraging that it often leads to more addictive behavior. Try any of these ideas to get back to safety.

o *If you lose, don't lose the lesson.* What's something new you learned that can help next time?

o *Identify the unmet needs.* Relapse means you wanted or needed something and didn't know how to satisfy that in some other way. Maybe you yearned for relaxation? Relief? Excitement? Connection with others? Understanding? Self-esteem? Listen closely to your needs and respond to them in healthy ways.

155

o *Notice something that's going right.* Even if it's just "I'm still breathing," hang on to that thin thread as if it's a lifeline. If you're still alive, there's something you did right. Notice what you still have, such as friends, family, a job.

o *Use survival skills.* Wilderness survivors (and you're in the wilderness when you relapse) say it's crucial to stay calm, keep your wits about you, figure out a plan, and stay hopeful that you'll find your way out of the woods.

o *Stop the bleeding.* Make the relapse as short as possible. It's like a tourniquet – quick first aid prevents further damage. Even if you relapse, how quickly you stop makes all the difference.

o *Understand that relapse is not an on/off switch; it's a dimmer switch.* It doesn't happen all at once (an on/off switch). Rather, it's a subtle set of signs that slowly increase in intensity (a dimmer switch). Signs include stress, boredom, irritation, tension, moodiness, and physical signs such as headache or stomachache. In the alcohol world, "BUD" is used to describe the build-up to relapse (<u>B</u>uilding <u>U</u>p to a <u>D</u>rink). Notice patterns unique to you. If you stay aware of these as they build you can respond better. Do *anything else* – work out, take a walk, play with a pet, call someone, watch a movie, and so on.

o *Do an instant replay.* Vividly picture the scene. What coping skills might have worked before, during, or after the relapse?

o *Bargain with yourself.* Delay self-blame for a while. Decide that if you can stop the behavior right now and get an hour/day/week clean, you won't hate yourself until the end of that time. This focuses you back on action rather than staying paralyzed in blame that just makes it all worse.

o *It's a fact.* Relapse is part of recovery for most people with addiction and trauma problems. At some point, one of their relapses was their last. This may be your last one too.

What to Do for a Relapse of *Trauma Problems*

Relapses of trauma problems are just as real as addiction relapses, and all the suggestions above for handling addiction relapse apply here too. But a relapse in trauma problems can be more subtle. There may not be clear behavior to observe, such as having a drink or drug. With trauma problems, you backslide to a "younger self," such as a childlike part of you that takes over with panic or fear. You may revert to a more paranoid state. Or you may feel unable to take care of yourself in mature ways.

✧ What does the opening quote to this chapter mean?

✧ What is one suggestion from this chapter that might work for you?

RECOVERY VOICES

Maggie – "My needs are valid."

Maggie survived childhood neglect and physical and sexual abuse. She has chronic pancreatitis from years of heavy drinking that began as a teenager. "Every time I know I have to go to the hospital due to an acute pancreatitis attack I become like a child again – a little girl. It's like I have these 'little ones' inside, clinging and desperate and scared. I throw tantrums (refuse to go); get 'bitchy' and take it out on my husband; think about ending it all or cutting myself (sometimes taking action); and feel panicky that this is the end. My husband, good friends, and therapist all work to help me come out of this state. Eventually I'm able to remember that I've been to the hospital many times, and each time I end up feeling better and can go back home. I carry a picture of my son to remind me of why I need to go in and take care of my body. I like that this chapter encourages me to stay aware of what I'm thinking, feeling, and wanting in the present. I have to remind myself that my needs are valid and real, and one way or another I can meet them or at least try to respond to them with compassion. My needs weren't met as a kid, so I can quickly flip into a young place where I have to yell to be heard. When I have a trauma relapse, I'm that kid again. I really believe I can learn to keep my adult self more present if I keep working on it. I was able to get abstinent from alcohol, which I'm so proud of, and now I'm working hard on my trauma issues."

24

See the link

Curiosity will conquer fear even more than bravery will.
—JAMES STEPHENS, 20th-century Irish novelist

Are trauma and addiction entwined in your day-to-day life? Seeing the connection helps you see why you do what you do. Becoming curious helps you go below the surface of initial reactions and frustrations.

✳ Explore . . . *The link between addiction and trauma in the present*

Step 1. Choose one behavior that you're doing too much, even if you don't view it as an addiction.

If you have more than one such behavior, repeat this exercise later for the other behavior(s).

Examples of behaviors: ▪ alcohol ▪ drugs ▪ shopping ▪ food ▪ gambling ▪ spending ▪ work ▪ exercise ▪ TV ▪ gaming ▪ self-harm ▪ sex ▪ Internet ▪ a sport or hobby ▪ pornography

What are your reasons for using _____?

Step 2. In **column 1,** check off current reasons for the behavior you listed above.

For example, if alcohol is a problem for you, are you using it *to get to sleep? to escape memories? to numb out? to be sexual?* Check as many in column 1 as are true for you.

Step 3. Now look at **column 2** for links to trauma.

Column 1	**Column 2**
To:	Example of link to trauma:
☐ Get to sleep	*Sleep problems are common after trauma.*
☐ Escape memories	*Trauma memories may feel too painful.*
☐ Feel more alive	*It can make you feel that you've "died inside."*
☐ Be sexual	*When sex is triggering, scary, or dull.*
☐ Hurt or punish myself	*To re-create trauma.*
☐ Rebel	*Against people with power over you.*
☐ Feel cool or popular	*When you feel like an outsider.*
☐ Express anger	*When the rage won't go away.*
☐ Fake a feeling	*To seem normal.*
☐ Connect with others	*When you're isolated.*
☐ Experience danger	*Because danger is so familiar.*
☐ Numb out	*When it's too hard to let yourself feel.*
☐ Get revenge	*Against someone who hurt you.*
☐ Relax	*When you're stressed or scared.*
☐ Forget about the past	*When it won't go away.*
☐ Get energy	*Because trauma problems sap your strength.*
☐ Feel close to a partner	*When real closeness is missing.*
☐ Commit slow suicide	*When trauma makes you want to die.*
☐ Seek thrills	*So excitement can make up for bad times.*
☐ Reduce symptoms	*Nightmares, flashbacks, tension, anger.*
☐ Reward yourself	*To make up for what you had to endure.*

Column 1	**Column 2**
To:	Example of link to trauma:
❑ Give up on life	*If it all feels just too hard.*
❑ Feel intensity	*When trauma has deadened you.*
❑ Feel good	*At least for a while.*
❑ Celebrate	*To feel joy for a change.*
❑ Have fun	*Because pleasure doesn't come easily.*
❑ Fill the emptiness	*When trauma creates a void.*
❑ Experience sadness	*When you can't cry.*
❑ Feel powerful	*Because trauma makes you feel powerless.*
❑ Decrease stress	*As in posttraumatic stress disorder.*
❑ Tolerate pain	*Of past or current trauma or its effects.*
❑ To remember	*If you have memory gaps about trauma.*
❑ Feel more	*When you feel detached, numb.*
❑ Feel less	*When you're overwhelmed by feelings.*
❑ Gain insight	*To figure it out when you feel lost.*
❑ Cope	*When each day feels like a struggle.*
❑ Be in your body	*If you dissociate.*
❑ Imitate someone	*Because you don't feel like enough.*
❑ Soothe	*Because you didn't get comfort from others.*
❑ Get away from your body	*When you dislike your body.*
❑ Get the job done	*To survive.*
❑ Other: _____	_____

✧ Any new insights?

✧ How did you feel as you did this exercise?

This chapter reinforces what you likely already know at some level: addictive behavior is a short-term fix that fades quickly. It doesn't resolve trauma in the long run. Honor your needs – if you have real trauma problems, you need real help. So too for addiction.

✧ What does the quote at the start of the chapter mean to you?

RECOVERY VOICES

David – "This helps me shift away from self-blame."

"I had tried numerous times to treat my addictions in isolation and my trauma in isolation. Sometimes I'd get better in the short term, but I was never able to sustain the positive change. The relapses with drugs and the trauma reenactments only got worse until I wasn't able to keep it together any longer. This chapter shows me how connected my trauma and addiction were. I really needed to stop using drugs because the drugs were fueling exhausting, dangerous trauma reenactments, but my trauma was fueling this belief that I was worthless and deserved bad stuff in my life. This chapter helps me shift away from the self-blame I was living under and instead work on developing skills to address both areas. I can move my recovery forward."

25

Practice

All life is an experiment. The more experiments you make,
the better.
—RALPH WALDO EMERSON, 19th-century American essayist and poet

Practice how you'd cope with difficult events. Pick from the scenarios in this chapter
or come up with others that are meaningful to you. Make it real and vivid – walk
through each step; picture what you'd think, feel, say, and do.

The more you practice, the more you'll be ready to cope with whatever comes
your way. Like an athlete picturing a golf swing in slow motion, get it into body memory. Be a coping athlete – don't let trauma and addiction win. Each time you cope well,
you build resilience.

Remember to choose good coping that doesn't hurt you or anyone else. For ideas,
see "Safe coping skills" (Chapter 12).

⭐ Explore ... *How would you cope ... ?*

- Your doctor finds a lump that needs testing.

- The court won't give you custody of your child because of your addiction.

- Your father puts you down in front of others.

- A date pressures you to have sex without protection.

- You're a veteran and overhear someone on the bus say the war you fought was
  a waste.

- You're in love with someone who doesn't love you back.

This chapter was adapted from *Seeking Safety* by Lisa M. Najavits (Guilford Press, 2002) with permission of
the author.

- A cop stops you for speeding and makes a racist comment.

- Your friends are invited to a party, but you're not.

- You find out your partner is cheating on you.

- A person who assaulted you is found not guilty in court.

- Your car breaks down, and you get a repair bill you can't afford.

- You're triggered by a news article that reminds you of your trauma.

- Your roommate isn't doing enough housework.

- Your child develops a serious medical problem.

- You're short on rent, and your friend offers an illegal way to obtain the cash.

- You gained 3 pounds even though you've been working hard at dieting.

- Your boss tells you your performance needs improvement.

- You're being harassed by your ex.

- Your wallet is stolen.

- A colleague keeps asking you to lunch and you don't want to go.

- You're trying not to drink but keep relapsing.

- A friend is always "busy" and can't get together.

- Your uncle who abused you will be at the family reunion.

- Someone cuts you off in traffic, almost hitting you.

- Thanksgiving is coming, and you have no place to go.

- You run out of your psych meds, and your doctor is out of town.

- Your mother says she doesn't believe you were sexually abused.

- A good friend tells someone else a secret you shared.

- You get turned down for a job you really want.

- Others? _____

Suggestions

Imagine it as a movie scene. Watch yourself coping as if you're the star of the movie. Or play the movie director who instructs the actor on what to do. Really imagine it.

Contrast safe versus unsafe coping. If the scenario is "Your doctor finds a lump that needs further testing," what would your *unsafe coping* be (getting high? panicking and assuming the worst?)? Next contrast what your safe coping would be (finding out as much information as you can? talking it over with a friend?).

Start easy. Build up to harder scenarios. This creates mastery, like a musician who practices simple scales and eventually plays complex songs.

Get feedback. This is important for any type of practice – athletic, musical, academic. A coach gives you realistic feedback while also encouraging you. Find people who can give you honest feedback on how well you're coping.

Remember the bottom line. Nothing – no matter what happens – has to lead to unsafe behavior. There is always a way to cope safely.

Make it fun. Find a coping buddy to rehearse scenarios.

Set aside time to practice. Learning fades if practice ends. Rehearse while you're walking, cooking, cleaning, driving, or any other routine part of the day.

✧ If you practice coping skills, how might your life improve – in a week, a month, a year?

RECOVERY VOICES

Barbara – "When you practice, you create new connections in your brain."

"I've been in therapy most of my life and have done a lot of trauma work. But I think another big part of my recovery has been just sheer practice. I role-play little scenarios in my mind – how I might say something to someone or how I'd think through something or coach myself through something. As the chapter says, it really is like an athlete doing all that preparation in sports psychology – picturing the scene, each move you'll make, and how you'll stay calm when there's havoc around you. I say to myself that it's like a muscle, and muscles aren't strong unless you practice. Like if your trauma involved the sound of gunfire and now you hear a loud explosion on the street, the way the neurobiology of trauma works is that you don't have a chance in hell to respond in a healthy way unless you practice. But when you practice, you create new connections in your brain and you have an alternative instead of spiraling down into unsafe addictive and trauma behaviors. That neurobiology piece is really important – it's there in your body until you retrain yourself to have a counterweight to those triggers. Both trauma and addiction are triggering, and I know that I need to do double-duty here and practice both types of triggers."

26

Identity: How you view yourself

All of the significant battles are waged within the self.
—SHELDON KOPP, 20th-century American psychologist

Who Are You?

This chapter is about identity: who you are and how you view yourself. The goal is to bring a compassionate lens to this core issue, one that takes into account how trauma and addiction play a role.

Arthur was sexually abused by a neighbor and later developed an alcohol problem. By the time he went into detox at age 36, his life was falling apart. He was on the verge of divorce and had to leave his job as an airline pilot due to alcohol. He was a kind and affable person but was very detached from his inner life: "For a while, I felt so far away – like I was on a big submarine off the coast, trying to get to shore. I kept getting flashes of my neighbor who abused me. I would wonder, 'Did I make all this up?' I was afraid to trust myself. For a while my own kids were a trigger. I wanted to drown out the thoughts with alcohol. It felt like nothing had a point. It's a lot better now. It feels weird to get in touch with myself and not be on guard. It's like a stranger."

Identity is your mental model of yourself. It's how you answer the question "Who are you?" There's no one way to answer it and, in fact, how you answer it says a lot about who you are. For example: "I'm 23 and in school. I'm friendly and outgoing but not really close to people. I grew up in Chicago but have lived in Austin for 4 years.

I'm first-generation American. I'm smart and attractive and like to read novels. . . . "
Or "I'm a college dropout who works as a proofreader. I'm a lot of fun when I'm not
depressed. I can't hold on to a job or a relationship. I'm really screwed up. . . . "

Who you are is a kaleidoscope of your age, gender, nationality, religion, ethnicity,
social class, temperament, relationships, how you spend your time, where you live,
what you value, what you survived, and so on. Identity goes to the core of your experience of life:

Identity [does] not mean only our noble features, or the good deeds we do, or the
brave faces we wear to conceal our confusions and complexities. Identity [has] . . .
as much to do with our shadows and limits, our wounds and fears, as with our
strength and potentials. Identity [is] . . . where all the forces that constitute my life
converge in the mystery of self: my genetic makeup, the nature of the man and
woman who gave me life, the culture in which I was raised, people who have sustained me and people who have done me harm, the good and ill I have done to
others and to myself, the experience of love and suffering – and much, much more.
—From *The Courage to Teach Guide for Reflection and Renewal* by Parker Palmer
    and Megan Scribner

✧ Not to impress anyone or to appear a certain way but, just within you, how
    would you answer the question "Who are you?"

✧ How would you describe yourself to others?

How Trauma and Addiction Impact Identity

Trauma and addiction may be as much a part of your identity as other aspects. They
influence you even if you don't want them to.

As in the quote from Arthur on the previous page, you may feel cut off from
yourself – unsure what you like and dislike, what you feel, what matters to you. Especially if trauma or addiction occurred when you were young, you may never have
developed a strong identity. You may not have been allowed to have your own point of
view. You may have had to grow up too soon, parenting your own parents or younger
siblings. You may have become numb, shut down, not feeling much at all.

You may also have a lot of strong feelings, but they're directed against yourself:

self-hatred and self-blame. You can do no right. There's a strong critical voice putting you down for just being you. The flip side of this dynamic is that you direct those harsh feelings toward others, usually someone weaker than you who can't stand up to you, such as a child or partner.

Trauma and addiction sometimes shift your identity in an instant. Combat may change you into a disabled amputee; driving under the influence may land you in jail. Suddenly you're part of a new world of hospitals or the legal system that wasn't part of your life before.

Another identity pattern is to become fully blended with "trauma victim" or "addict." You may feel you *are* these rather than they are problems you have: "I'm a junkie" rather than "I'm someone with a heroin problem." At the other extreme you may negate aspects of your identity that are true. You may say, "My trauma wasn't really that bad," even though you are isolated in the house, afraid to go out; or "Everyone says I have an addiction, but I don't."

It's also common to flip back and forth between extremes: "I'm fine/I'm a mess"; "I have a future/My life is over"; "I can fix this/It's hopeless"; "I didn't deserve it/It was all my fault." As you work on recovery, you'll find greater wholeness – a more consistent view of yourself and one that's larger than trauma and addiction.

Finally, both trauma and addiction are associated with *splitting*, which is a fragmented identity in which you're only aware of part of yourself at a given time. A classic example of splitting in addiction is referred to as *Jekyll and Hyde* (from the famous book by Stevenson): one side of you wants to keep using, the other side wants to recover. In trauma, splits also occur. At times, you may be aware of only one side of you, such as a young side or an angry side. Everyone has sides they're aware of at different times, but in trauma and addiction the splits tend to be more extreme, less conscious, and more likely to lead to unsafe behavior. With recovery comes integration – balanced awareness of all sides of the self and greater control over them.

✧ How have trauma and addiction affected your view of yourself?

Use Who You Are to Promote Recovery

Some aspects of identity are more fixed, such as age, gender, and ethnicity. Others are more malleable. For example, personality traits are part of your identity and can be expressed in healthy or unhealthy ways. Usually the unhealthy version is too extreme or directed toward unworthy goals.

To enhance your recovery, take such aspects of your identity and steer them toward healthy expression.

Unhealthy version of self	Healthy version of self
People pleaser; too concerned with how others view you	A people person, able to connect, values others
Perfectionistic, obsessive	Focused on quality, detail oriented
Low energy, lazy	Laid back, easygoing, low drama
Critical, judgmental	Perceptive, observant
Impulsive	Spontaneous
Manipulative	Engaging, charming, strategic
Cheap, withholding	Independent, values security
Angry, vengeful	High energy, sensitive to right and wrong, strong sense of justice

This is not just rewording – saying what's bad is good or flipping a negative to a positive. It's about accepting who you are and directing the traits that define you so they don't cause problems but instead become a source of your success.

Example. Laura is a college student who sees herself as "perfectionistic and obsessive" when she's under stress. She spends far too much time worrying about small matters and then feels bad about herself for not getting her work done, which leads her to isolate and engage in severe food binges.

But when she's able to take better care of herself (taking breaks, setting clear goals to keep her work on track, getting sleep, spending some time with people instead of constantly alone), she views herself as "focused on quality, detail oriented"; these are positive traits that help her succeed in school. She is still who she is, but this part of her personality has a healthy versus unhealthy version that she can bring out. The idea is to direct aspects of your identity to lift you up rather than drag you down.

✧ Is there a personality trait that you can mold into a healthier version?

How Your Identity Changes with Recovery

In successful recovery, you learn to tell a new story of who you are. You become the hero of your story.

» From victim to survivor

» From silence to finding your voice

» From powerlessness to a sense of control

» From isolation to connection

» From hidden to known

» From fragmented to whole

✧ How would it feel to shift your identity in these ways?

✧ What aspects of your identity are you most proud of?

✧ Do you see yourself as the *hero of your story*? If not, how might you gain that perspective?

RECOVERY VOICES

Sarah – "Now my recovery identity is pretty strong."

Sarah has years of successful recovery from childhood trauma, substances, self-harm (cutting), shopping addiction, and anorexia. "I'm years into recovery from trauma and addiction, and *identity* is still something I'm working on. Some of the other parts of this book I had moved beyond, but this topic I'm still very much working on – it's a huge deal. When I look back on it, I've tried five major identities. The first was 'religious Catholic girl'; it started in fourth grade, when I was in Catholic school. I went all out, way beyond my peers. I made my own Eucharist to take to the priest and have it blessed and then brought it home and kept it in my closet. I was super-intense about Catholicism for a couple of years, until my family decided to do an exorcism on me, and I never went back to it after that. Then I started using drugs heavily and didn't have a clear identity until my next one, which was a 'Cambridge atheist bookworm.' That was a very strong identity and worked well with the Cambridge people. Then it was a 'religious orthodox Jew'; and then it was 'mental patient' – I went into the hospital a professional, functioning person and came out carrying a teddy bear, regressed; this was in the 1990s. After that I transitioned to suburban housewife. That's been the hardest of all; I've hated it the most, but it's been the safest. This question of identity is something I go over every day. I feel this tiny quiet voice of myself now, but it's still small and weak. I feel it when I do yoga or when I'm really calm. Maybe identity is something most people start building in childhood, but that didn't happen for me. The inner life I built was a response to the horrible external life events that were going on – I was just focused on surviving, not building an identity. I went from one addiction to another, totally numbing out. I really think a lot of it was to get away from these kinds of questions about identity. If you face your inner life without something to numb out, it's really freakin' hard to do until you learn how. My mind would keep seeking ways to get away, to not have to cope with all the stuff that was flooding in. But now my recovery identity is pretty strong. It's not a solid state; I'm still challenged throughout the day, but when I come up against challenges I'm able to choose the recovery identity most of the time, even if it's hard. Like when a flashback comes I used to get sucked into the drink, the pills, the cutting, to feel what seemed like comfort. But now I find other ways to deal with it that are more enduring, more real. In this chapter where it says, 'Who are you?' my answer is 'I'm small but very strong.' I'm like a compact mass of matter with a lot of energy."

27

Perception: How others view you

We are all apt to believe what the world believes about us.
—GEORGE ELIOT, 19th-century British writer

Do you have major concerns about *how others see you?* Many people with trauma and addiction are subject to negative perceptions by others, directly or indirectly. It may have a name such as "the crazy sister," "the junkie," "the trigger-temper veteran," "the black sheep of the family." Even if you don't have a name for it, you may have a sense of it in some way, feeling that you're seen as tainted, bad, weak, or dangerous.

In healthy, supportive environments the same process happens, but in the opposite direction. The image people hold of you would be positive, such as "the go-to person," "an old soul," "the brains of the family." They would see you as a valued member of the group, a good person.

You likely have a mix of both positive and negative images that others *project* onto you – that come from them.

Trauma, Addiction, and Social Perception

It's hard enough to deal with trauma and addiction, but if there's an added layer of negative social perception it's even tougher.

Trauma and addiction are two of the most stigmatized emotional problems. You may feel rejected, blamed, or scapegoated for having them. It's as if others aren't really seeing you; they're seeing a caricature, an all-or-none concept of who they think you are. You're a problem or embarrassment to them and you can't shake those perceptions no matter what you do.

Erving Goffman, a social psychologist, describes three categories of people:

1. Those who are *stigmatized.*

2. *Normals* who aren't stigmatized.

3. The *wise normals* who understand and accept the stigmatized: "Wise persons are [those] before whom the individual with a fault need feel no shame nor exert self-control, knowing that in spite of his failing he will be seen as an ordinary other."

Historically, and still today in some cultures, people who suffer trauma such as rape are blamed and shunned for it. Or the trauma survivor may be feared rather than supported.

Addiction is stigmatized too. Even doctors, health professionals, and sometimes other addicts judge people with addiction harshly. Negative social perceptions of trauma and addiction can occur in any social environment – work, school, the criminal justice system, the health care system, and within families and communities. Even after you're on a good recovery path, it may feel like you're never forgiven for the past, never given a fresh start.

Although some people may hold unfair negative perceptions of you, there definitely are people out in the wider world who don't. There are caring, wise people who understand trauma and addiction; it's just a matter of finding them. And just as important, it's about strengthening your ability to rely on your own truth – what you know to be good about yourself.

◇ Do you believe that you're unfairly seen as tainted (bad, weak, or dangerous)?

◇ Do you feel that you can "do no right," that some people see you in a negative light no matter what you do?

◇ Do others' perceptions of you feel painful or disturbing?

◇ Do you have some traits that some people interpret positively and others negatively (e.g., you're very sensitive and some people value that and others put you down for it)?

"The Reign of Error"

Beyond trauma and addiction, you may have other features that people automatically react to negatively without getting to know you: a disability, homelessness, HIV or other illness, history of criminality (even if you served your time), mental illness in your family, sexual orientation, race, gender, ethnicity, or your job (e.g., sex worker).

It's been cleverly called the *reign of error* because it's such a distortion of reality. It views members of a devalued group as being all the same. There's no longer a person there – just a trait or part of your history that they fear or dislike.

It occurs in every society and across history. One explanation is based in evolution: people distance from those they perceive as weak, who may be seen as a threat to survival. It also occurs when people can't own their weaknesses and instead turn against others (the "kick the dog" phenomenon).

An Example

Military personnel with PTSD suffer multiple layers of stigma. During military service, they may be perceived as weak if they seek counseling; they were trained to be "tougher than that." After they leave the military, the public may view them as a ticking time bomb, liable to burst into crazy violence. If they have addiction, that adds yet more stigma.

Employers hesitate to hire veterans due to such perceptions. Yet the reality is that most veterans don't physically harm anyone, and if they do they're far more likely to hurt themselves via suicide than to be violent toward others.

C. J. Grisham served in Iraq as an Army sergeant. He developed PTSD from combat, including being forced to shoot someone being used as a human shield. His PTSD included flashbacks, depression, and suicidal feelings. There were "a million voices in my head telling me that I'm not good enough to be alive." He felt weak for being depressed and selfish for surviving when his friends didn't. He had intense anxiety: "I get extremely nervous in crowded situations. . . . Before entering any building, I make a quick survey of all people around me and seek out any and all exits. I sit with my back to a wall so I have a good view of people approaching me. I get startled and anxious at unexpected and loud noises. What I don't get is violent. What I don't do is threaten people."

—From "U.S. veterans struggle with pain, stigma of posttraumatic stress: New research aimed at mental health," by Charlotte Tucker in *The Nation's Health*

Becoming Who They Say You Are

Some people absorb the negative perceptions so deeply that they live them out. This phenomenon has various names, such as *self-fulfilling prophecy, self-stigma, enacting the projection,* and, a related term, *the soft bigotry of low expectations.* It's as if there's a script created for you and you act it out, except that it's all too real. Maxine Harris and colleagues, who interviewed traumatized women with substance abuse, describe it poignantly:

"A number of women described feeling defeated by the weight of their past bad choices. Using drugs and alcohol had become a way of life that, although it had its obvious negative consequences, also had a certain predictability that left a woman feeling oddly comfortable . . . using drugs was an accepted and expected way of life within their families. More than half the women reported that relatives not only used drugs but sold them and that the family elders expected that girls in the family would eventually use drugs and enter the sex trade to support their habits. Some women even commented that mothers, cousins, or aunts who were already involved in the drug subculture introduced them to drugs and prostitution. In such families, news that someone had achieved sobriety was met with derision and scorn. . . . Finally, some women talked of being addicted to the drug culture itself. For these women, the activities that accompany addiction had an allure of their own."
—From "Special section on relapse prevention" in *Psychiatric Services*

If you've lived out the negative expectations of others, you may find it hard to see yourself in a new way, such as "I'm a good person," "I can make a difference," "I can succeed," "I can be a good parent," "I can find healthy relationships." But you *can* learn new strategies to live out these positive identities.

What to Do

Negative perceptions by others can feel like a force field of overwhelming power. You need strong ways to fight it. Try any combination of the following ideas.

Distance

Creating distance from people who project negative images onto you can give you the emotional space to figure out who you really are independent of them. It can be physical distance, such as entering rehab or moving away, or psychological distance, such as not engaging in discussions that tap into their negative image of you. Distance buys you time to become different.

✧ Would it help to create distance from people who don't understand you?

"Play in a New Sandbox"

Find new people who can see you as you are today, without the weight of the past. They can be a powerful presence to reinforce your best self and to appreciate the future you're trying to build.

✧ How can you find new people who can see you in a new light?

Notice Double-Edged Traits

Take a new view of traits that others have criticized in you. For example, if you're very sensitive, some people may see that as weakness, but it can also be seen as highly aware and artistic. See "Identity: How you view yourself" (Chapter 26) for more on such double-edged traits.

✧ Try looking at your traits from both sides.

Reinforce a New Perception of Yourself

Gain ground by holding on to a new view of yourself. It's like a mantra or a TV ad that replays over and over: "I'm someone who copes with whatever comes up," or "I'm a person who's patient rather than someone who yells." See "Create a healing image" (Chapter 31) for more on how to expand an image like this.

✧ What is a new perception you'd want to reinforce?

Create a Second-Act Plan

Develop a clear vision of your best possible self. This is sometimes called a *second act*: the first part of your life was Act I, and now you're the writer and director of Act II, the next segment. Rather than accepting the script others gave you, write a vision of what *you* want. It's also called *reinventing yourself.* The key is it must be realistic so you can achieve it.

> ✧ What is your second-act plan? Picture it, write it down, draw it – anything to bring it to life.

Live Out the New Plan

An essential part of overcoming negative perceptions of you is to actually *be* different. It can't be just words – your new image must be visible by your behavior in the real world. Even if other people stick to their views, you get better at holding on to your truth and not stepping back into the behaviors that prove them right. Use all the tools you can to achieve and maintain your new identity.

> ✧ How will you live out your new plan? How will your actions be different?

Find Role Models

Look for examples of people who have overcome stigma. Explore among people you know, in books, and online.

> ✧ Do you know any inspiring examples of people who reinvented themselves?

Join with Others to Promote Social Justice

Consider joining an organization as an advocate or volunteer to help others who are stigmatized. Make use of your difficult experiences in positive ways. See "What the wounded can give back" (Chapter 34).

> ✧ Would it help you to join with others to fight stigma?

RECOVERY VOICES

Gina – "I remind myself to remember the truth."

Gina was emotionally abused and has struggled with food and marijuana addiction since her teen years. "I always felt I was good for nothing and whatever I did seemed to never be good enough. I was told that many times, and it felt like it was just a given. I remember early in my life realizing that whenever I cared about something the people in my life would use it to make fun of me or they would take it away from me. I had to learn not to care about anything. As a result, I got really good at being good at nothing and not caring about anyone, and one day I realized that I now saw myself the same negative way my family had always seen me. I was 14 years old. This chapter helps me look at this in a way I hadn't quite done before; and in my group therapy I've learned that others have the same kinds of experiences. That really helped me see how a child who was told she was no good would end up agreeing with that, like I did. But now that I'm more aware of how the process works I remind myself to remember the truth – that I was a good kid and I was good at some stuff.

"It's interesting to read about the three types of people: 'the normals, the stigmatized, and the wise normals.' It gets me out of feeling like it's just *me* that's the problem. Even as an adult in my family I'm still seen negatively – 'the crazy one, no good.' But for the most part at this point I wouldn't do much different, which is partly why they get frustrated with me; they still want me to believe their version of reality. I just see things differently than they do. I love the paragraph about how some people see you as a caricature, all-or-nothing, a problem. Ding! That's exactly what it feels like. I'm going to have to work on this topic for a long time, because it's so hard to hang on to positives about myself. I've made progress, but it's still too easy to fall back into harsh one-sided judgments that mirror what they said about me all those years. If I gain weight or mess up on something, I call myself names, and that drives me even more into negative behavior. I'm planning to work various parts of this chapter, especially trying to surround myself more with people who accept me and see me in a positive light."

28

The decision to grow

Have patience with everything unresolved in your heart and try to love the questions themselves as if they were locked rooms or books written in a very foreign language. . . . And the point is to live everything. Live the questions now. Perhaps then, someday far in the future, you will gradually, without even noticing it, live your way into the answer.

—Rainer Maria Rilke, 20th-century German writer

This chapter is about becoming a student of life. Even if you were never especially good at school, you can become an outstanding student of life itself. Notice the natural world, which is always growing, with changing seasons, births, deaths, and renewal. So, too, you can keep growing emotionally; and the more you grow emotionally, the stronger your addiction and trauma recovery will be.

Emotional growth is, above all, a *decision*. You may feel so worn out that you've given up. Your world may be narrow, focused on physical survival, just existing. You may no longer care what happens. You may go through the day shut down, cut off. Yet no matter how low you feel, you can *always* make the decision to grow. People with even the most severe trauma and addiction have found within them, in a moment of inspiration or despair, that decision to grow. It's saying yes to life, yes to just trying.

The musician Pablo Casals was 95 years old when a reporter asked, "Mr. Casals, you're 95 and the greatest cellist who ever lived. Why do you still practice 6 hours a day?" Casals said, "Because I think I'm making progress."

What Did You Learn?

In trauma and addiction you learned all sorts of lessons, even if you weren't aware of them. It's important to respect that you adapted to your environment. You did your best to survive. But as the saying goes, "What got you here won't get you there." The goal now is to expand your learning to what will best promote recovery.

With *trauma* you may have learned:

▪ "Don't trust." ▪ "Pretend nothing happened." ▪ "It's best not to feel." ▪ "You're no good." ▪ "People will take advantage of you." ▪ "The truth can't be spoken." ▪ "It's safest to be alone." ▪ "No one will protect you." ▪ "Don't bother trying."

With *addiction* you may have learned:

▪ "Don't worry about tomorrow." ▪ "This is the way to escape pain." ▪ "I like myself more when I'm using." ▪ "It gets me through tough times." ▪ "I only feel close to people when I'm using." ▪ "Nothing matters." ▪ "I can't keep promises."

In *healthy environments* people learn lessons such as:

▪ "Stay away from dangerous people." ▪ "Be yourself." ▪ "Conflicts can be handled without violence." ▪ "There's help out there if you look for it." ▪ "You're a good person." ▪ "You can make progress if you put your mind to it." ▪ "Everyone makes mistakes." ▪ "Take good care of your body." ▪ "Build trust with safe people."

◇ Circle any messages above that you learned.

New Learning Can Improve Brain Functioning

Addiction and trauma, in addition to the direct suffering they cause, can impair learning and brain function. Both can affect concentration and memory, making it harder for you to retain information. They can reduce judgment and abstract reasoning, leading to impulsive decisions that don't serve you in the long run. They can alter your ability to react, sometimes dulling your reactions and other times leading to overreactions. Such brain changes usually occur below the level of awareness.

But with new learning, the physical structure of the brain changes and you can improve in multiple areas, according to research.

✷ Explore . . . *Encourage yourself to grow*

People who recover quickest and best are those who are able to peek out from behind their old learning and ask, "Is this serving me now?" and "Will this help me recover?"

In school, you learned subjects like science, math, history, and literature. Now you can decide what topics matter to you.

This exercise offers a simple set of steps to encourage yourself to grow. Later it will become more automatic; you'll naturally keep learning.

Question 1: What do you want to learn?

Anything can be learned. For example, you may want to learn how to . . .

- Find real friends

- Manage cravings

- Say "no" to protect yourself

- Get along with people who are different from you

- Respond to someone who puts you down

- Coach yourself through tough times

- Calm yourself when you get upset

- Engage in sex that's safe for you

- Find a job

- Create new habits like healthy eating and exercise

- Keep your promises

- Stay safe

- Get organized

- Increase your motivation

Others have learned these topics, and that means you can too. They likely had healthier environments that gave them a better start. But the essence of recovery is that you can learn at any point and live out the best version of yourself.

List here any topics you want to learn. You can choose from the list above and add in others.

_____

_____

_____

_____

_____

Question 2: How do you learn best?

There has been a lot of research on how people learn.

One approach focuses on *learning styles,* emphasizing different pathways of learning (visual, written, verbal, and physical touch learners). Another approach focuses on *independent* versus *group* learning. Another addresses *top-down* learning (based on reasoning) versus *bottom-up* (learning from experience). *Multiple intelligences* conveys the idea that there are different types of intelligence: mathematical, linguistic, social, musical, and physical as well as *emotional intelligence,* which is a gift for understanding one's own and others' feelings.

More research is needed to verify these theories, but they convey an important point: there are different ways to learn.

You can increase your learning by figuring out *how* you learn best. Experiment with as many of the following learning methods as you can:

- Talking with others.
- Searching on the Internet (search using any of the topics listed in Question 1, such as "How to find real friends" or "How to get organized").
- Reading (self-help books, etc.).
- Writing (try keeping a journal on a topic you are trying to learn).
- Taking a class or joining a group to learn with.
- Watching videos (see "The world is your school," Chapter 6).
- See the resources in this book (Appendix B).

The goal is active learning – doing all you can to engage with experiences and conversations to move forward. Learning is an active process, not a passive one.

How do you learn best? Describe here how you'll go about learning any of the topics you chose in Question 1.

_____

_____

_____

_____

_____

_____

Question 3: What motivates you to learn?

In addition to *what* you learn and *how* you learn, be prepared for feelings that arise. Learning can bring up fear, excitement, feeling stupid, feeling smart, and a lot else. Know that it's all normal.

Sustain your motivation by . . .

- Doing what you can to push forward, however small

- Getting feedback from others about how you're doing

- Looking for lessons wherever you can find them

- Being patient with yourself; no one gets straight A's at life

- Tolerating confusion and uncertainty

- Trying to enjoy learning at least some of the time

- Accepting that learning is a struggle at times

- Being compassionate when things don't go well

- Making an active effort rather than just drifting along

- Caring about the results

- Keeping your heart open to what you're learning

- Tolerating awkwardness: the stumbling and false starts

- Knowing there's always more to learn – and that means there's hope

What motivates you to keep learning? Draw from the list on the previous page and add your own . . .

_____

_____

_____

_____

_____

All of life is an experiment; grow from new experiments each day.

> ✧ From 0 (not at all) to 10 (extremely), how committed are you to new
> learning? If that number is low, how can you increase it?

> ✧ What are examples of new learning that have helped your recovery?

RECOVERY VOICES

David – "It's okay to feel uncomfortable and awkward."

"This is one of the most challenging topics. For me, it's about doing things out of my comfort zone. Drug use and trauma reenactments, while incredibly painful and destructive, had become my norm. They were essentially my comfort zone. When I was sober, I was uncomfortable and felt awkward. My home had become drugs and unsafe behaviors. I like that this chapter reminds me that it's okay to feel uncomfortable and awkward. I need to challenge myself every day to do something different. In sobriety, I like to exercise, and the way I get my muscles to grow is by pushing them to a place of discomfort. I think it's the same with emotional growth. The drugs and trauma fill me with fear, but if I push myself to try new things and am okay with failing, I think the fear will dissipate over time and I'll grow stronger. For me, the keys to learning are to practice compassion, to be gentle with myself, and to try something new – something small but new – every day. What I have found is that with time, experience, and sobriety comes clarity and slowly, very slowly, wisdom, and then, ultimately, humility. The thing about recovery is the longer a person is in it, the less 'wiggle' room he has with the bullshit negative behaviors. I still watch too much TV at night as an escape and also look at porn at night – not every night, and with the porn not the way I used to – but instead of getting 8-plus hours of sleep I get 7 or less on some nights because of those behaviors. The next day I get into work late and don't have as much inclination to take care of paperwork that needs attention. So what does that mean? Well, that I am human and have opportunities for growth. I exercise regularly, meditate daily, eat well, pray throughout the day, get more sleep than ever before, connect regularly with positive friends, do my best to be of service at work and to help the people whose paths intersect mine – and all these things I do quite imperfectly."

29

Dark feelings: Rage, hatred, revenge, bitterness

Feelings have their own kind of wisdom.
–NANCY McWILLIAMS, American psychoanalyst

Trauma and addiction can evoke dark feelings such as rage, hatred, bitterness, desire for revenge, and sadism. You may have your own language for them – cruel, monstrous, ugly, unforgiving, vengeful, furious, spiteful.

"I had not learned about pain without wanting to inflict it. I had not endured torture without wanting revenge."
—Survivor of the Cambodian genocide, in *Haing Ngor: A Cambodian Odyssey*

"I carried this home with me. I lost all my friends, beat up my sister, went after my father. I mean, I just went after anybody and everything. Every three days I would totally explode, lose it for no reason at all. I'd be sitting there calm as could be, and this monster would come out of me with a fury that most people didn't want to be around. So it wasn't just over there. I brought it back here with me."
—Vietnam veteran, in *Achilles in Vietnam: Combat Trauma and the Undoing of Character*, by Jonathan Shay

---

✧ Do you have intense anger outbursts?

✧ Do you have a lot of thoughts about revenge?

✧ Do you resent people who seem happy?

✧ Do you feel stuck in bitterness?

✧ Do you want to get rid of such feelings but can't?

✧ Do these feelings take a toll on your life?

Everyone has these feelings at times, but with trauma and addiction they may be so intense and out of control that they scare you or others. You may try to suppress them but then get triggered and explode. You may be obsessed with endless-loop thoughts of revenge. You may feel angry at everyone and everything. You may be ashamed of your dark feelings but have no idea what to do about them. People may say, "Stop thinking about it" or "I don't want to hear it," leaving you alone with what's inside. You may direct the dark feelings at yourself as well as others.

Dark feelings have a magnetic pull. And for some people they're more than a metaphor; they represent a dark physical place where these feelings arose – a prison, a basement, or a crack den. The feelings can be paralyzing, preventing you from moving on. Yet if understood, they can be directed toward healing. They are important feelings to pay attention to.

The Many Versions of Anger

Many dark feelings are rooted in anger that has mutated into an unhealthy form. Hatred is a deeper, more extreme version of anger. Bitterness is anger mixed with helplessness. Rage is explosive anger. Contempt is anger turned into putdowns of other people. Sadism can be wanting others to feel the hurt that you feel. The term *anger* is used in this chapter because it's at the core of many other feelings, but choose whatever language fits for you.

Your Feelings Make Sense

Dark feelings are there for a reason. You may want to get rid of them as if they're a cancer to be cut out, but anger isn't bad in and of itself. It's built into the biology of humans as protection against predators in the wild. Anger is like a country's army: it gets called up to fight when there's a threat. Respect that it's there to protect you. In fact, not being able to feel anger can keep you just as stuck as too much anger. But when anger is too persistent or too intense, it's not healthy.

Steve said, "My father used to hit me when he was drunk. When I was 15, I decided to fight back. I didn't want to fight my own father, but I needed to feel that he couldn't totally dominate me. It helped me survive. But it's made it hard to be in close relationships, because I instinctively fight when there's a problem – a lot of yelling and sometimes it gets physical, which I'm not proud of. I haven't figured out how to get along without fighting."

✧ On an average day, how much of your time is taken up with dark feelings?

Responding to Dark Feelings

The goal is to *respond* to your dark feelings. This means you use active methods to transform your relationship with them; you become less consumed by them.

Responding also means that you don't go to unhealthy extremes: too little or too much. "Too little" is when you ignore or suppress the dark feelings; then they burst out anyway in some form, such as blowing up or impulsively hurting yourself or others. "Too much" means you let out their full force without any filter; but this gets out of control and is dangerous.

Redirect the Energy

If you direct the energy in your dark feelings toward healing, it can bring you to healthier emotional states.

Michele writes, "I used to be angry at my own PTSD suffering. I used to be angry my trauma happened in the first place; no one shielded me from harm; no one could stop the horrific event from continuing. . . . On a bad day, I could add to my already deep depression with a powerful dose of anger and then – watch out! I was really a sight to behold. That depressive anger I usually turned inward came out with a ferocity that flayed anyone around me. I feel sorry for the people I directed it at, particularly my family. But 7 years ago this New Year's Eve I decided to take that angry energy and use it in a positive way: I decided to pursue joy and . . . it worked! All of that antsy angry energy spilled onto the dance floor and out of me. I became more peaceful, more tolerant; less angry, more . . . well . . . happy. Being angry at others is . . . time and energy that we really need to be channeling toward healing. Using that energy on ourselves can bring relief, so we shouldn't so easily give it away."

—From Michele Rosenthal, *PTSD & Anger, Part 1: When We Hate Happy People*

✧ How can you redirect your angry energy?

Let Yourself Grieve

Trauma and addiction come with many losses: loss of hope, innocence, trust, physical integrity, money, relationships, and freedom. You may have no idea how to grieve these. A survivor of child abuse said, "Growing up, if I was upset my parents would say 'Go to sleep and when you wake up your problems will be gone.'" As Jonathan Shay wrote in *Achilles in Vietnam*, during the Vietnam War, "Mourning was dreaded, perfunctory, delayed, devalued, mocked, fragmented, minimized, deflected, disregarded, and sedated." Underneath dark feelings there are often deep layers of hurt and sadness. Release those deeper feelings to convert your anger to a less toxic form.

Become Curious

Explore your patterns . . .

○ *Are you* addicted *to anger?* Rage can be a habit just like other addictions. Revenge fantasies can have an addictive quality – obsessing about them and spending too much time on them. If you're addicted to anger, there's usually some degree of pleasure in it; it feels good in the moment, powerful and righteous.

○ *Is anger part of substance use or withdrawal?* Cocaine, methamphetamine, and other drugs can create out-of-control paranoia and rage.

○ *Is anger part of a medical illness?* Anger and rage attacks can be caused by overactive thyroid, traumatic brain injury, dementia, autism, and other conditions. Sometimes these go unidentified for years.

o *Does anger relate to early messages you learned?* Stuffing anger or being demeaned or punished for it can make it grow stronger, like a weed that pushes up through the concrete.

o *Are you part of a subculture that values anger?* For example, gangs live by violence and intimidation. Once you're in that culture it becomes normal.

o *Do you have major ongoing stress?* Erupting in anger may be a cry for help or a way to vent when stress puts you over the top. Trauma and addiction are stressful, and there is often added stress from unemployment, divorce, poverty, bullying, discrimination, and loss.

o *Is anger a way to feel heard?* If you believe that others don't understand you, anger may be a way to try to be heard. But they may listen less because they feel scared of you.

o *Does anger take you by surprise?* It may take over without warning. For example, some military veterans lash out physically at a partner in their sleep, never intending to.

o *Are you mirroring what was done to you?* You may erupt in hatred or rage in ways that mirror how you were treated.

Whatever the reasons for your dark feelings, staying curious about them can reveal new ways to work on them. For addictive anger, you can take strategies you're learning about addiction recovery and apply those to anger too. If your anger is based in stress, you can find better ways to manage stress. If you have a medical condition, you can seek help for it. If anger takes you by surprise, you can learn greater awareness. And so on.

◇ What are your anger patterns?

Find a Mission Greater Than Your Rage

People with dark feelings are often highly idealistic, valuing respect and fairness. Trauma and addiction erode these ideals, but you can rekindle them by finding some important mission. This is the basis for AA, Mothers Against Drunk Driving, domestic violence shelters, rape crisis programs, homelessness programs, and nonprofits of all kinds that have been created and nurtured by people in recovery from trauma or addiction. Pursuing a meaningful goal also creates distance between you and your dark feelings, which helps reduce their too-strong hold over you. You lose perspective when caught up too strongly in dark feelings; a life mission can bring that back. See "What the wounded can give back" (Chapter 34) for more about helping others while reinforcing your own recovery.

✧ What goal is more important to you than your dark feelings?

Learn Flexibility, Like an Athlete

If you're stuck in feelings, you need to gain flexibility. Just for an athlete, it takes a lot of practice, coaching, and exercise to develop that. With dark feelings, learn how they build up, how to coach yourself through them, how to shift out of them, how to be with others without letting the feelings take over. Find people who do it well and learn from them. Keep learning new, flexible methods.

✧ How flexible are you with your dark feelings?

Protect Others from Your Rage

Dark feelings such as rage can be scary to others, especially those close to you. Once you're in that zone you're no longer "you" – you're in a primitive brain, closer to a wild animal than your best self. You may feel justified, but your perception has narrowed to where you can't be reasonable and fair; you can't see another person's point of view.

So try to prepare ahead of time, while calm, for what others should do if you get that way. This keeps them safer and helps you preserve important relationships. If there's no preparation, they may cower, try to appease you, or lash out, which can incite your anger even more.

One idea is to create a code word or phrase that allows them to distance if they need to, such as "I need to be on my own right now" or just a word like "safe." Then they can go to another room, out for coffee, or to any other safe place. This lets them set a boundary for self-protection, and it buys you time to calm down. Other plans can be developed based on the type of relationship and your own patterns. There might be a time limit in which you talk (but not yell) about your feelings and then stop; this prevents an endless retelling of gripes that reinforces rather than relieves the dark feelings. Another option is to collaborate on preparing a sequence of easy, low-key calming activities to do together such as watching TV or taking a walk but with no discussion of what you're angry about until your feelings come down. Working with a couple or family counselor may help too.

✧ Can you try any of the ideas in this section?

Learn from Revenge Fantasies, but Don't Act on Them

Revenge fantasies are a sign of unmet needs. They can be a source of growth if you handle them the right way. There are three basic steps.

1. *Be clear that you can never act on the revenge fantasy in any way that would actually damage someone.* Fantasies are normal, whether they are about revenge, sex, or wish fulfillment, for example. Everyone has fantasies. But acting on them in any way that is unethical, illegal, or causes physical or emotional damage is never acceptable. Acting on a revenge fantasy, moreover, keeps you bound up with people who hurt you; it robs you of time; and it reinforces your powerlessness by keeping you stuck in a victim–perpetrator dynamic. It can also lead to jail and other real-world consequences.

2. *Explore the underlying needs in the fantasy.* Typical needs in revenge fantasies include:

» Wanting to have power over others or render them powerless.

» Having others feel the pain that you felt.

» Wanting others to acknowledge what they did to you.

» Getting an apology.

3. *Find ways to get your needs met in the present.* There's no way to change the past, but you can find healthy, real ways to get your needs met now rather than focusing on the fantasy.

Mike was physically abused by his father and then bullied and humiliated by an older boy in middle school. "I want to find that kid now and set his house on fire. I'd leave a message in black char with the word 'fag' on it, which is what he tormented me with in school." Mike went as far as researching where the man lived and how he would do it, which scared him.

Mike opened up to his counselor about the fantasy. They established that they could talk honestly about it but it could never, ever be acted on (step 1). Then they worked to identify Mike's underlying needs (step 2): he wanted to feel respected rather than humiliated, powerful rather than powerless, and to have his sexuality accepted.

Mike worked with his counselor to brainstorm ways he could feel respected and powerful now (step 3). They tried having him rehearse in his mind standing up to the boy, creating a new ending to what happened back then. They tried having Mike become a "big brother" volunteer to a middle-school boy who was being bullied. They worked on writing a letter to the man who had bullied him, though they didn't mail it. Mike also began to work out to feel physically stronger; and he and his counselor explored how he had been affected first by his father's abuse and then by the bullying. The combination of these helped to lessen the intensity of his revenge fantasy by directing his energy back to the present in growth-oriented ways.

◇ Do you have revenge fantasies? Can you go through the three steps either alone or with someone you trust?

If There's Danger of Violence, You Must Get Help

If you're in danger of harming yourself or others, it means you're not able to manage your feelings on your own. Call a hotline, go to an emergency room, make an appointment with a counselor – whatever ensures that you're not alone with the darkness that has taken over. It will get easier if you get help.

RECOVERY VOICES

Brad – "I try really hard now to take responsibility for my feelings."

"I served three tours of duty in Iraq, and by the time I returned to civilian life I had a truckload of rage. That actually worked for me pretty well in the military for what I had to do. But when I came back, I saw the toll it took in everyday life. My friends stopped hanging with me; but the worst part was what it did to my wife and kid. Even though I never hit them, I could see fear replace the love that had been there. Behavior that felt so instinctive for me in the military was destroying my family. It dawned on me that I would scar them like I'd been scarred. My father was in the Army in World War II and came home a rageaholic; I didn't want to become like him.

"This chapter reminds me that I'm not the only one who deals with feelings like this and that there are some ways out. So what do I do now? Anything and everything! I see the rage as part of my PTSD, and I can't let it devour me. I've also come to see my rage attacks as an addiction just like substance addiction, and that's helped me too. The biggest part of my growth has been to accept my flaws but to own my actions. I try really hard now to take responsibility for my feelings rather than directing them toward whoever's in my path. I'm still triggered, but I try to remember that I can either choose to bully those around me or just try to relax in the face of stress and handle it without blowing up. Sometimes I walk away so I won't take it out on people. I see the efforts my wife makes, and I love her for that, and I love my kid unconditionally. His lifelong happiness will depend on the choices I make, just like mine were by my dad's. These days my family still sees a somewhat sullen and depressed man, but the love is starting to replace the fear in their eyes, and that means the world to me."

30

Imagination

Everything you can imagine is real.
—PABLO PICASSO, 20th-century Spanish artist

One of the best tools to bring to recovery is your own imagination – playing with possibilities and envisioning what isn't yet present. Imagination moves you past inner defenses that keep you from your full range of feelings. It taps into wisdom you didn't know was there. You discover fresh perspectives that can spur growth.

Studies show that imagination promotes wellness. Imagination-based games have been developed for many health conditions and show positive impact on disease outcomes. Such "serious games," as they're called, tackle physical and mental illnesses through playful methods including avatars, immersion in pretend worlds, and made-up quests and missions. In highly engaging ways, they remind people to take medication, manage chronic illness, and improve diet and exercise. Creativity is also identified as one of the eight primary methods that produce psychological transformation in "How do people change?" (Chapter 5).

This chapter uses imagination to help you gather resources for addiction and trauma recovery – skills, tools, strategies, supports, inspiration – anything that sustains you. The exercise is designed to be playful, so have fun with it.

⬩ Do you have a childlike side that enjoys play?

✳ Explore . . . *Play with your recovery imagination*

Here in Part 1, let the exercise drift over you, picturing it in your mind, feeling it. Linger in sections you like and shift away from what you don't respond to. You don't need to do anything else.

Step 1: *Imagine you have a huge container filled with recovery resources*

The resources are many shapes, sizes, and colors, and there are so many that you need a huge container to hold them. Your container is perhaps a big lake . . . a sports stadium . . . a box the size of a house . . . or a set of shelves that go from the floor to the sky.

Step 2: *Step closer and look inside your container*

There are five recovery resources, each focused on one key question.

(A) THE INSPIRATION BOOK: *WHAT INSPIRES YOU?*

The *inspiration book* has illustrated pages like a glossy magazine, a scrapbook, or the illuminated manuscripts of medieval monks. The pages have inspiration for recovery – quotes, prayers, poems, mantras, songs, proverbs, drawings, humor, and stories. As you skim the pages you feel lighter and stronger. The pages are decorated, perhaps with glitter or calligraphy, and are made from artistic paper, fabric, or an antique scroll. The book has your initials on the front and a lock to protect it.

(B) THE SAFETY NET: *WHAT KEEPS YOU SAFE?*

The *safety net* catches you if you start to fall. It's like a spiderweb – thin and light but extremely durable. The more time you spend spinning the web, the stronger it becomes. The safety net holds a lot, including phone numbers to call when you're in trouble, hotlines, emergency rooms, shelters, and treatment programs. Safety is a central task of recovery: keeping yourself as physically and emotionally safe as possible. Imagine safety – what would it look like in your life?

(C) THE GO-TO ACTIVITY KIT: *WHAT BRINGS YOU JOY?*

The *go-to activity kit* has joyful activities to enliven recovery: dancing, humor, games, movies, sports, music, and more. The kit is like a child's dream with activities for home and outdoors, warm and cold weather, and any time.

(D) THE HEALING IMAGES COLLECTION: *WHAT IMAGES SUSTAIN YOU?*

The *healing images collection* is a shortcut to your deepest ideals. Visual images can remind you of what matters. Are you a warrior battling the forces of addiction with a sword? Are you a detective noticing facts and clues to understand your trauma? As the writer Milan Kundera said in *The Unbearable Lightness of Being*, "A single metaphor can give birth to love." See "Create a healing image" (Chapter 31) for more on finding images that are meaningful for you.

(E) THE BACKPACK OF RECOVERY SKILLS: *WHAT SKILLS MATTER TO YOU?*

The *backpack of recovery skills* is the learning you carry forward from support groups, treatment programs, self-help books, and life experience. It has worksheets, exercises, and skill reminders like "Surround myself with positive people," "Try delaying the drink," "Structure my day to stay focused," "Use grounding when triggered," and "Call a friend for support." These are in your backpack so they're close by when you need them. You can fill the recovery backpack with all sorts of skills: bits and pieces that may help a little or big, bold recovery skills that will take you far. It's valuable, so don't lose it.

Step 3: *Notice how you feel*

Take a moment to notice how you feel. Engaging your imagination typically evokes brighter, lighter feelings. It's creative – an open-ended adventure that feels *alive*. Amid the ups and downs of recovery, imagination can be a positive force.

Step 4: *Transform your imagination into action*

Now the goal is to construct real recovery resources if you choose to. Take one or more of the five described in Step 2 and start working on its *form* and its *content*. Remember that each is a collection of some kind to help support your recovery.

Form. This means its container, a place to store the recovery resources you're creating. Choose something that's easy for you to get to so you can return to it easily. Make it big enough so you can keep adding to it over time.

Examples: ▪ a scrapbook ▪ a box ▪ a bag ▪ a folder on your computer ▪ an electronic collection (e.g., Google Drive, Dropbox, Evernote, Pinterest)

Content. Now the idea is to put as much as you can that is meaningful to you into the recovery resource. You may already have some material to start with and/or may want to embark on a search. Here are some examples of ways to find good content.

(A) THE INSPIRATION BOOK: *WHAT INSPIRES YOU?*

Go online or visit a bookstore or library to find recovery-related quotes, prayers, poems, mantras, songs, proverbs, drawings, humor, stories. Write out a vision of what you want your life to look like in 3 months, 6 months, a year. On your phone, record yourself or others offering encouraging statements. Write a journal about your recovery insights. Write a list of your strengths (and, if helpful, weaknesses to remember too).

(B) THE SAFETY NET: *WHAT KEEPS YOU SAFE?*

Find phone numbers and addresses for local emergency rooms, treatment centers, and shelters. List hotline numbers (suicide hotline, domestic violence hotline, etc.). Find self-help meetings in your area. Write a list of people you can call. Start a list of reasons for living. Develop a safety contract with a counselor. Write a letter or create a voice recording now from your "best self" to remind you why and how to stay safe.

(C) THE GO-TO ACTIVITY KIT: *WHAT BRINGS YOU JOY?*

Find fun things: dancing, humor, games, movies, sports, music. Try new recipes. Explore local fun activities by scanning newspapers and *meetup.com* groups. Join a club. Take classes to learn a new sport, language, or craft. Go on daytrips or weekends away. Search online for "how to find fun things to do."

(D) THE HEALING IMAGES COLLECTION: *WHAT IMAGES SUSTAIN YOU?*

Images can be photographs, drawings, or any other visual object. Find beautiful photos such as nature scenes. Keep close some photographs of people who inspire you, including people you know and famous people. Take pictures of objects that are meaningful to you, such as a beautiful stone or an AA chip. Find images that represent life goals you can achieve with successful recovery: a healthy body, a new-born baby, a university degree. If it helps, you can also collect images that represent the dark side of recovery to remind you of what you want to avoid (e.g., graveyard, hospital, overdose).

(E) THE BACKPACK OF RECOVERY SKILLS: *WHAT SKILLS MATTER TO YOU?*

There are many ways to find skills. In this book, see "Safe coping skills" (Chapter 12) and "Getting to a calm place: The skill of grounding" (Chapter 18). Go to a library or bookstore and browse the self-help section. Ask others what skills they use. Search online using terms such as "trauma recovery tips" and "ideas for addiction recovery." Collect worksheets and other recovery materials at treatment and self-help meetings.

Step 5: *Embrace the resources in your daily life*

Use your recovery resources every day, even if it's just for 3 minutes. Look through them so that they seep into your consciousness. If possible, do it the same time each day, such as while making coffee or before going to bed.

Keep expanding them. The more you add, the more valuable they become. They are your nest egg, your riches. They help you live the life you want.

✧ "Recovery is a creative process" – what does that mean to you?

RECOVERY VOICES

Sophie – "I was able to imagine leaving."

"I grew up in a house full of lies – lies that were told to me and that I was forced to tell to people outside the family. That's what kept the whole system going. We were like the cast of a play with scripts that kept us from talking about what was really happening, like my father's alcoholism and all the trauma that came from that. From when I was very young I knew that I wanted to get out of there as soon as I was old enough. I think that's what helped me survive a really sick family – that I was able to imagine leaving. My sisters couldn't; they stayed and suffered hugely for that. Staying was a key part of the script: 'blood is thicker than water, the family has to stay together, you can't survive on the outside,' and so on. My family is all still there, and their lives are miserable, with addiction and trauma in the next generation with my sisters' kids. I was the only one who left. I always knew I had to get out of there. I didn't know what I was going toward, only what I wanted to get away from. There was no game plan, no blueprint. No one in my family helped me apply to college, but I figured it out with a teacher's help and left at 18. I think my imagination saved me from becoming like them. I don't know why I could picture leaving, but I know it was clear to me. As a kid I pictured the bus pulling out of town, the fields disappearing into the background (we lived on a farm), and images like that. I'd return to those images again and again and took comfort in them. What I really like about this chapter is that it expresses how important imagination is. I haven't heard it talked about like that before, but I've seen in my own life that if you can use your imagination for recovery it can help you do what you need to do. The practical part of this chapter also appealed to me: that imagination is put toward creating something physical, something real – the recovery resource. I've always had an artistic streak, and I get a lot out of this type of exercise. I worked on the inspiration book as my recovery resource. I've spent several hours on it and want to keep going. I think it'll help keep me grounded, and it validates the recovery work I'm already doing. It can also mark my progress. I'm putting a date on each page so the book becomes a chronicle of healing; I'll be able to look at it a year out and see how far I've come by looking at the pages. The inspiration book is a way of telling the truth about how I see things. It's an antidote to the lies I grew up with."

31

Create a healing image

When the image is new, the world is new.
—GASTON BACHELARD, 20th-century French philosopher and poet

Visual images are powerful and can direct your mind and body toward healing. Imagery is now used in medicine to help people get through childbirth, cancer treatment, chronic pain, and other physical challenges. Research shows that healing imagery decreases physical pain and helps people recover faster. Positive images lower your heart rate, decrease stress, and improve digestion. Negative images have the opposite impact. Images can also improve performance. Musicians who imagine playing a piece of music strengthen their ability to play it. Athletes who visualize a game do better on the field.

Notice How Images Make You Feel

Explore how you respond to images. Some people are naturally stronger visualizers than others, so just observe your reactions. There's no right or wrong.

✧ Try this simple exercise.

1. Picture as vividly as you can an image that's *inspiring* to you. It might be a beautiful, strong horse galloping in a field or a springtime graduation (can you hear the music? do you see caps tossed into the air?). Really see it for a few moments and notice how you feel in your body and heart.

2. Now picture an image that's *unpleasant* for you. It might be gridlock traffic

(you're late for work, and now this!) or rain ruining a picnic. Same thing here: really see it for a few moments and notice how you feel in your body and heart.

3. Do you notice a difference between how you feel with image 1 and image 2?

Healing Images for Trauma and Addiction

Now let's apply the idea to trauma and addiction.

✧ Notice how you feel as you read these images.

» *Protection*: a suit of armor, ancient city walls

» *Escape*: airlifted out, rungs of a ladder

» *Love and nurturance*: a bird building a nest

» *Fighting back*: a magic shield, sword, battleship

» *Connection*: a circle of people dancing

» *A new life*: sculpting clay, a baby

» *Transcendence*: a rocket, a secret passage to safety

✧ Can you come up with other inspiring images related to trauma or addiction?

The rest of this chapter guides you to create an image to reinforce your recovery. It can bring you back to what's most important. Choose an image that relates to both trauma and addiction if you have both. The image can be a photo, a drawing, or a physical object. Some examples:

Judy chooses "a photo of my baby daughter": "When I look into her eyes, I see myself in her and say, 'I can do this.' She inspires me to keep doing what I need to do. She gets me to go to treatment when I don't want to."

Margo chooses "a hot-air balloon rising into the sky": "To me, recovery means I can get beyond my awful past and sail into a bright sky. When I look at the picture, it inspires me to rise up – to get off the couch and get some exercise and take better care of myself."

Dave chooses "the logo of the school I want to get into": "If I can get into that school, I feel like I have a chance. I don't want to keep dealing drugs and stealing; those are crazy-dangerous. When I look at the logo, I snap back to reality and start planning my day to move things forward."

Notice in each example that there are three parts:

1. An image
2. A personal meaning that promotes recovery
3. Specific recovery actions

✶ Explore . . . *Create your healing image*

Answer these four questions to create a strong recovery image. An example is provided after the questions.

Question 1: *What recovery image will you choose?*

_____

_____

Question 2: *What meaning does it hold for you?*

_____

_____

Question 3: *What recovery actions will you take based on it?*

_____

_____

Question 4: *How will you make your image ever-present?*

_____

_____

Example

Question 1: *What recovery image will you choose?*

"An Olympic swimmer."

Question 2: *What meaning does it hold for you?*

"I'm a recovery athlete. I need to have a lockstep routine every day so that I practice hard, build my body, and keep my mind sharp to compete and win."

Question 3: *What recovery actions will you take based on it?*

"I'll follow my recovery routine every day, whether I feel like it or not, just like the swimmer who gets in the pool and does laps against the clock each morning. I'll refuse any substance that's offered to me. I'll get myself to my appointments. I'll get enough sleep. I'll stop hanging with people who use and/or distract me from my goals."

Question 4: *How will you make your image ever-present?*

"A photo of the Olympic podium with the banners and crowds. I'll load it as the wallpaper on my phone so I'll keep seeing it."

Carry It with You

Make the image ever-present in your heart by creating reminders of it:

- Load it onto your device (phone, tablet) as wallpaper.
- Place it around your home: on a nightstand, refrigerator, etc.
- Put it on an object such as a keychain photo.

RECOVERY VOICES

Marta – "Not living in a fantasy"

"I grew up seeing a lot of violence by my dad toward my mom, and there was nothing I could do to stop it. I've had several relationships where I was abused, too, starting as a teenager. Now I'm committed to finding a healthy partner. Reading this chapter, I decided to work on an image to get me more in touch with my feelings. Usually, I'm so focused on the other person that I have no idea what I want, and I end up in bad relationships, feeling hurt or scared. I find myself shutting down when there's any conflict or disagreement. The image I chose is a thermometer, the old-fashioned kind with the red mercury that rises up the hotter it gets. I'm trying to notice how I feel with different people, like my boss, my mother, my friends. I'm trying to identify times I feel valued and respected versus times I feel uncomfortable or unsure of what's happening, not listened to, or mistreated and controlled. I like the thermometer image because it's simple and it helps me notice how good or bad I feel with different people. When I feel relaxed and comfortable, the thermometer is low; when I'm tense, the thermometer goes up. I use a funky retro image of a thermometer as wallpaper on my phone to remind me. Little by little, I'm more able to see what's really happening in the moment – not living in a fantasy of what I want to happen. It's a big step for me to become aware. I feel more hopeful about finding a healthy relationship."

32

Find a good counselor

"My counselor is like a cup of warm tea on a cold winter day."

"My doctor gave me answers I was looking for. I don't feel so crazy now."

"After I see my therapist I want to drink."

"My counselor accused me of abusing my daughter by drinking. I never went back."

At some point many people with trauma and addiction find themselves in counseling of some sort. It's important to find a helper who's a good fit for you: someone who's supportive yet also guides you to make real changes in your life. A good professional helper is more than a kind friend; it's someone who:

» Sets clear goals.

» Understands and monitors your symptoms.

» Gives you honest feedback.

» Provides options.

» Uses methods that produce results.

» Knows how to handle emergency situations.

» Keeps you on track.

» Helps you feel safe so you can say anything without feeling judged.

This chapter was adapted with permission from *Creating Change* by Lisa M. Najavits (forthcoming from The Guilford Press).

Trauma and addiction create unique challenges in finding a good counseling relationship. If you grew up in an unstable environment, you may be so hungry for a positive parental figure that you stay too long in a treatment that isn't working. Or the opposite: you may be too quick to leave when difficult feelings arise rather than learning new ways to handle them.

You also need someone knowledgeable about trauma and addiction.

"Professionals need to know how to deal with people's despair, fear, anxiety, grief, rage/anger, cutting, suicidal thoughts – not make them feel guilty for feeling it or respond with 'Oh, you shouldn't feel that way.'"
—From *In Their Own Words: Trauma Survivors and Professionals They Trust Tell What Hurts, What Helps, and What Is Needed for Trauma Services*

Addiction requires expertise too. Signs of lack of expertise include not asking you about addiction at all, not monitoring your level of use, conveying demeaning attitudes ("once an addict, always an addict"), and using old-style harsh confrontation. A good helper will balance support and accountability, provide options, and inspire you to become the best you can be in relation to both your trauma and addiction. And, crucially important, a good counselor will not violate boundaries or get defensive if you give feedback. Also the counselor should be flexible and willing to try other strategies rather than persisting with what isn't working for you.

Unfortunately, there are too many stories of unhelpful counselors. One woman said her counselor told her to write a letter of forgiveness to her trauma perpetrator or she would "never recover." Another said, "My counselor used to be really negative toward me. He seemed to dislike me and if I had a slip and drank he'd tell me I was 'treatment-resistant and noncompliant' and 'lacked insight.' I never felt supported by him." Yet when done well, counseling can be extraordinarily helpful, even life-saving.

Like most things, the quality of counseling ranges from excellent to poor. And easy-to-measure counselor characteristics have almost no connection to how good a counselor is. For example, none of the following predict how well counselors do with their clients, according to research: the counselor's age, gender, ethnicity, number of years of experience, type of degree, cost, or being in recovery themselves. People with "Dr." in front of their name (PhDs and MDs) are, on average, no better than counselors without these degrees. So, too, the counselor's own history of trauma or addiction can be a strength or weakness, depending on the person. Even a counselor who comes highly recommended may not be a good fit for you in terms of personality or your specific issues. In a *New York Times* article titled "After PTSD, More Trauma," a Marine officer described how he got worse, including increased alcohol use, while in the care of a Veterans Affairs therapist who was more intent on sticking to a PTSD therapy protocol than truly listening to him.

How can you tell who's a good counselor for you? There's a simple yet reliable way to evaluate whether your counseling is likely to be helpful in the long run. It's called a *helping alliance scale,* and it allows you to rate the quality of your counseling experience. Such scales have been tested based on extensive research. Remarkably, ratings by the third session of counseling predict how helpful it's likely to be months and even years later. The exercise in this chapter offers a scale you can use.

Your Part

Even with the best counseling, you need to do the work of showing up, trying new things, being open to feedback, and following through on tasks. Recovery is yours to create. But it's likely to go better if you have someone on your side who you trust and feel can help you. Invest in yourself by finding someone who's a good fit for you. Some people spend more time shopping for a smartphone than for a good counselor.

Know too that it's normal, especially in long-term counseling, to have a range of feelings toward your counselor, including admiration, anger, appreciation, disappointment, and closeness. Good counseling provides a safe place to talk through these feelings to help you grow. The more intense your trauma and addiction issues, the more likely it is that your relationship problems will show up with your counselor as well. A good counselor helps you see those patterns and deal with them constructively.

✶ Explore . . . *Evaluate your counseling*

The questionnaire on the next pages is research tested and reprinted here with permission. If you're in counseling now, fill it out based on your current counselor. If you're not in counseling but willing to try it (a good idea – the more help, the better), you can "shop around" and meet with several different counselors, using the scale to help you decide which one to continue with.

The Revised Helping Alliance Questionnaire –
<u>Client Version</u>

Instructions: Carefully consider your relationship with your counselor and then mark each statement according to how strongly you agree or disagree. Please mark every one.

A *counselor* refers to any counselor, therapist, or other professional helper who holds sessions with you to address emotional issues and life problems. Circle one answer in each row based on the wording at the top: how much you agree or disagree with each statement. Don't focus on the numbers; after you finish, there will be instructions for scoring your answers. Also, remember that the scale is not rating you (your problems, your progress). There are no right or wrong answers.

Name of the counselor you're rating: _____

	Strongly disagree	Disagree	Slightly disagree	Slightly agree	Agree	Strongly agree
1. I feel I can depend on the counselor.	1	2	3	4	5	6
2. I feel the counselor understands me.	1	2	3	4	5	6
3. I feel the counselor wants me to achieve my goals.	1	2	3	4	5	6
4. At times I distrust the counselor's judgment.	6	5	4	3	2	1
5. I feel I am working together with the counselor in a joint effort.	1	2	3	4	5	6
6. I believe we have similar ideas about the nature of my problems.	1	2	3	4	5	6
7. I generally respect the counselor's views about me.	1	2	3	4	5	6
8. The procedures used in my therapy are not well suited to my needs.	6	5	4	3	2	1
9. I like the counselor as a person.	1	2	3	4	5	6
10. In most sessions, the counselor and I find a way to work on my problems together.	1	2	3	4	5	6

From Luborsky et al. (1996). Reprinted with permission from the American Psychiatric Association.

	Strongly disagree	Disagree	Slightly disagree	Slightly agree	Agree	Strongly agree
11. The counselor relates to me in ways that slow the progress of the therapy.	6	5	4	3	2	1
12. A good relationship has formed with my counselor.	1	2	3	4	5	6
13. The counselor appears to be experienced in helping people.	1	2	3	4	5	6
14. I want very much to work out my problems.	1	2	3	4	5	6
15. The counselor and I have meaningful exchanges.	1	2	3	4	5	6
16. The counselor and I sometimes have unprofitable exchanges.	6	5	4	3	2	1
17. From time to time, we both talk about the same important events in my past.	1	2	3	4	5	6
18. I believe the counselor likes me as a person.	1	2	3	4	5	6
19. At times the counselor seems distant.	6	5	4	3	2	1

Scoring. Make sure you have an answer for each question, then add the total of all the items you circled. Scores range from 19 to 114. The higher your score, the more you feel helped by your counselor. If your score is high, that's great. A total of 85 or below indicates that you have a poor alliance (you don't feel helped enough by your counselor) and suggests a need for further action. You can try talking with your counselor about it (highly recommended), asking people you trust for feedback, and reading further in this chapter.

The scale was changed as follows: the terms *therapist* and *patient* were changed to *counselor* and *client*; the scale's reverse scoring was incorporated into the layout for simplicity; minor grammatical errors were corrected; and the instructions were expanded.

Keep in Mind . . .

o *Every counseling relationship has ups and downs.* A particular session may not be useful or you may feel out of sync with your counselor. That's normal and can even be a source of growth. A poor alliance is an ongoing feeling about the counseling, not a brief dip from the usual pattern.

○ *Counseling can be warm and supportive, but should not feel like just chatting with a friend.* The time should be heavily focused on specific strategies, exploration of important themes in your life, and attention to deep feelings. If your counseling feels consistently superficial or chatty, look elsewhere.

○ *Studies show that clients' ratings of the helping alliance are a better predictor of progress than counselors' ratings of it.* So trust your ratings and your own perceptions.

○ *Get feedback from people you trust.* With trauma and addiction, you may doubt your own point of view and feel confused. Seek input from multiple people. Also, you can obtain a formal consultation by a counseling expert, although you usually would have to pay for that.

○ *Shop around.* If you have the option to try out different counselors, do so and then decide who's best for you. You can try a few sessions with each before deciding. See "12 questions to ask when seeking help" in "Find your way" (Chapter 9) for ideas on what to ask. If you're mandated to treatment (required to attend, such as by a court), you may not have a choice of counselors. But even in such situations, you can sometimes ask to work with a different counselor as long as you stay in treatment.

○ *Counselors should never violate professional ethics.* This includes all sexual contact, financial improprieties such as insurance fraud, or violating your confidentiality. You can report such issues to your state licensing board. If a counselor initiates sexual contact of any kind, stop seeing that counselor immediately and get help elsewhere.

○ *Talk openly with your counselor to work out problems that come up in your relationship, but set a reasonable time frame for it.* And don't stay in a treatment out of guilt or emotional pressure by the counselor. Counseling is supposed to help you; you're not there to meet the counselor's emotional needs.

○ *It's normal for counseling to bring up painful feelings and feel difficult at times.* This doesn't mean something is wrong, as long as you believe the counselor is helping you work on these.

○ *Research shows that the counselor is more important than the type of counseling (the "brand name").* But if a counselor is using a specific counseling approach, you have the right to know the name of it and its evidence base (whether it's been scientifically tested) so that you can look it up and learn more about it.

○ *Remember that the* Helping Alliance Questionnaire *is evaluating your perception of your counseling.* You also can benefit from other questionnaires that measure your addiction and trauma problems to see whether you're improving over time. See "Resources" (Appendix B) to find such measures.

○ *Search online.* Learn more by searching terms such as "helping alliance," "how to find a good therapist," "how to decide if your therapist is good," and "how to tell if therapy is working."

○ *Read more in this book.* Other chapters that focus on treatment include "Find your way" (Chapter 9), "Two types of trauma counseling" (Chapter 33), and "It's medical – you're not crazy, lazy, or bad" (Chapter 4).

✧ If you're currently in counseling, is there anything from this chapter that you'd like to share with your counselor?

✧ Are you able to speak openly with your counselor about any topic? If not, what might help build greater trust?

RECOVERY VOICES

Karla – "I've seen it all – the best and the worst counselors."

"I've seen it all – the best and the worst counselors. I've been in counseling since I was a teenager due to multiple sexual assaults and problems with food and alcohol addiction. One would get angry with me when I became suicidal. He'd say, 'Just use the coping skills you were taught.' He didn't get it that I would use the coping skills if I could, but when I'm in another state of mind, full of despair and self-loathing, it isn't always so easy. I needed help to figure out how to remember the coping skills and to use them in dark moments. I also had counselors who were terrific, although there were a lot fewer of those. My favorite, who I saw for years, was amazing. No matter what I brought up, she found a way to work on it. She helped me see parts of me that were good when I couldn't see them myself. I started to feel there were things worth living for. If I was triggered and having horrible memories of my vulnerability when I was so young and sexually abused, she was patient and we worked on those but without her ever pushing too hard. When I had relapses, she hung in there while other counselors would tell me that I wasn't motivated enough or that I was 'sabotaging myself' (whatever that means). She also taught me practical skills, and that made a big difference in how I handled my day-to-day. She was able to really hear me. I've found that good counselors are empathic and accept what you say as your truth, as far as you know it. The other ones filter it through their own life experiences rather than reacting to what you're saying. They judge rather than understand.

"It's also important to know that there's a lot of power in a counseling relationship. When I didn't feel safe in counseling, I was always worried about angering my counselor or protecting myself from my counselor's wrath or indifference. I had one who kept going off on me, yelling at me. No one should have to deal with a counselor yelling at you. There are also practical issues to think about. I've been in clinics where we get churned through one after another because the counselors were on a 6-month rotation. It's hard to keep starting over with someone new. What I like most about this chapter is that it's very real about what goes on. Too often I've felt like I was the problem if counseling didn't go well. This chapter has a nice way of showing that it's a two-way street; the client and counselor each have to do their part. I also liked the questionnaire, which is a great tool for how to think about therapy. I wish I'd had this chapter way back when. It's not easy to find a good therapist; I think they're few and far between. My advice to others would be to keep looking until you find someone you can trust."

33

Two types of trauma counseling

Be not afraid of growing slowly; be afraid only of standing still.
—Chinese proverb

Trauma counseling can be a wonderful option if you have trauma problems. But many people are hesitant to start because they don't understand that they can choose different ways to go about it. You may be surprised by what you'll discover in this chapter.

◇ If you like quizzes, try this one now or when you finish this chapter. Either way, keep reading . . .

1. "Trauma counseling means you tell your trauma story (what happened) in detail."
   True / False
2. "You have to reduce your addictive behavior before you work on trauma."
   True / False
3. "You need to tell your trauma story to recover fully."
   True / False
4. "If you feel ready to tell your trauma story, you're ready."
   True / False
5. "You can work on addiction and trauma at the same time."
   True / False
6. "After you tell your trauma story, your addiction will go away."
   True / False
7. "The more intense the trauma counseling, the more you'll recover."
   True / False

The answers, with explanations, are at the end of the chapter.

Present- versus Past-Focused Trauma Counseling

There are different "brands" of trauma counseling, but they come down to two basic types: *present*-focused and *past*-focused. Each can be helpful, or you may want to try a combination.

Present-Focused Trauma Counseling

> Fall down seven times, get up eight.
> —Zen saying

Present-focused counseling is a practical "how-to" treatment that teaches you coping skills to manage current trauma problems.

You can learn how to manage trauma triggers; how to leave damaging relationships; how to respond to yourself compassionately when trauma problems arise; how to shift feelings when they're too much (overwhelming) or too little (numbing); how to express yourself to get your needs met; how to reduce unsafe behavior such as addiction; how to take better care of your body; how to build good relationships; how to create new meanings to counter trauma beliefs ("I'm defective"; "People will always hurt me"). You explore how trauma impacts your current life – your relationships, thinking, and behavior – and improve your ability to cope in healthy ways.

Just as important is what's *not* done in present-focused trauma counseling. You're not asked to tell your history of trauma in detail. You might choose to share briefly about the nature of your trauma, but you won't be asked to explore painful, vulnerable details. The focus is headlines, not details: you might say, "I was sexually abused as a child," but you wouldn't be asked to go through the long version of it (exactly who did what, how often, what you felt at the time, etc.).

There are various present-focused trauma models, including *Seeking Safety, present-centered therapy, trauma recovery and empowerment, stress inoculation training, cognitive therapy, imagery rehearsal therapy, beyond trauma,* and *trauma affect regulation: guide for education and therapy.* Another widely used present-focused coping skills model is dialectical behavior therapy, but it wasn't developed for trauma/PTSD and is not yet evidence based for that (Harned, Korslund, & Linehan, 2014). Also most present-focused trauma models were not designed for or tested on people with addiction. The most researched and evidence-based model for people with both trauma problems and addiction is Seeking Safety (*www.seekingsafety.org*; details are in "Substance Use Disorder and Trauma" in Najavits, Hyman, Ruglass, Hien, & Read [2017], *Handbook of Trauma Psychology*; see References).

Present-focused models are helpful for people who want to get better but don't want to explore intense trauma memories, or at least not right now. They prefer to learn how to cope in the present. Present-focused models can be done in individual or group counseling and anyone can participate in them; they're extremely safe.

Shelly describes how she worked on trauma and addiction using a present-focused model, Seeking Safety: "It saved my life. I don't know how to say it strongly enough. It turned my life around. The idea that *you're* the agent of safety in your life and that's what's going to save you *is* what saved me. I became aware of my choices and concrete steps that I could do even when it felt like there was nothing I could do. My therapist and I worked on all kinds of safe coping skills: setting boundaries in relationships, taking better care of my body, learning how to ask for help, making commitments toward my recovery, developing compassion toward myself, and so on. The results were almost immediate, and it made me want to do more. Over time, I developed the language and the feeling and the experience of safety. My life was so filled with tragedy and excruciating pain that it felt like those were never going to go away. But I gradually rebuilt my life, brick by brick, into one far better than I had thought possible. I feel joy now. I've found a few people who love me. And when problems come up, I know at a gut level that there are ways to deal with them rather than escaping into drugs, fantasy, hurting myself, food, or any of the old stuff I used to do. I guess the therapy gave me what kids get when they grow up in healthy families but which I never had. I still have work to do and likely will for the rest of my life, but I know I'm on a path of growth."

Past-Focused Trauma Counseling

To get to the healing you have to break your heart first.
—Dorothy Allison, American novelist

In past-focused models, you explore your trauma story in detail to "work it through." You learn that you can sit with trauma memories and feelings, tolerate them, and eventually they no longer hold such emotional power over you. You grieve the past so that you can be at peace with it. You don't forget that trauma happened, but you're able to come to a deeper sense of acceptance that allows you to move on with your life.

There are many variations on past-focused models. Some ask you to tell your trauma story out loud; others have you write it; and in some you explore it in your mind but you don't say it out loud. As you delve into your trauma memories you may be encouraged to observe what you feel in your body or to notice beliefs you hold about the trauma ("It was my fault"). You might explore themes related to trauma such as intimacy, power, or silencing. You might be asked to look at reminders of trauma either in the therapy or as homework, such as reading a news article about it or going to a place that reminds you of it. Some models use techniques such as eye movements (back-and-forth visual tracking) to help you process your trauma. What all these models have in common is a paradox: you're encouraged to move into painful trauma memories and feelings as a way to overcome them. Most past-focused trauma models are done in individual counseling, although some can be done in a group.

Past-focused models arose with Sigmund Freud in the 19th century and go by many different names, in the modern era, including *testimony therapy*; *eye movement desensitization and reprocessing*; *exposure therapies (e.g., narrative exposure therapy, prolonged exposure therapy, written exposure therapy)*; *virtual reality therapy*; *cognitive processing therapy*; *abreactive ego state therapy*; *accelerated resolution therapy*; and *emotional freedom techniques*.

It's important to know, however, that past-focused models were designed and primarily tested on people who did *not* have additional serious problems such as addiction, homelessness, domestic violence, suicidal/violent impulses, head injury, serious physical health problems, or major mental illness such as psychosis or bipolar disorder. Past-focused models were considered too intense for people with these sorts of problems. In recent years, there have been some attempts to adapt past-focused models for people with co-occurring addiction, but thus far studies don't show any better results than for less emotionally intense, present-focused models. The field is still young, however, so future research will help clarify these issues. Also, some people with trauma problems and addiction do benefit from past-focused models.

Daniel used a past-focused model for trauma and addiction called Creating Change: "The best aspect of this therapy was that I understood early on that I was the one who would have to take the supplied tools and apply them. It was difficult to go back into my mind and memory and revisit the multiple traumas, but the therapy taught me that up until now I was revisiting it with the mind of a ten-year-old. The therapy taught me to see it with the mind of a 38-year-old. This completely changed my perception of the abuse and I was freed of shame and responsibility. The work is arduous and painful and it is only the desire to be well that got me through it. Dealing with the past and substance abuse was not only fine, but it allowed the substance desire to be less powerful. Since it was the PTSD that drove the substance abuse, it makes perfect sense to address them simultaneously. I can't thank you enough. You saved my life."

—From Lisa Najavits, *Creating Change*, in Ouimette and Read (2014)

Combining Present- and Past-Focused Trauma Counseling

You may benefit from trying each type (if you're able to do that) and then choosing what fits best for you. Or you can combine them. For example, you could start with present focused and then do past focused, or do both at the same time (perhaps present focused in group therapy and past focused in individual therapy).

There has been very little research, however, on combining them. Some studies evaluated models that are designed to include both present- and past-focused elements (*brief eclectic psychotherapy*; *concurrent treatment of PTSD and SUD using prolonged exposure*; *skills training in affect and interpersonal regulation/exposure*; *trauma management therapy*; *dialectical behavior therapy for PTSD*; *resilience-oriented treatment for PTSD*; *integrated cognitive-behavioral therapy for PTSD and alcohol use disorder*). Surprisingly, there is not yet any evidence that combining present- and past-focused elements does better than either one alone. Here, too, more research is needed.

More . . .

Both Types of Counseling Work

You may hear some people say that past-focused models are the best, the most powerful, or the "gold standard." Or they may convey inaccurate messages such as "You *must* tell your trauma story to recover." Many people believe that because past-focused trauma counseling is more emotionally intense than present-focused it must produce better results. But research shows that both types of treatments work without notable differences between them. The bottom line is that you have choices, so pick what fits for you.

It's Typically Best to Start with Present-Focused Trauma Counseling

Experts in trauma counseling agree that *safety* is the first stage of trauma. Present-focused trauma counseling is often a good choice at the start to ensure that you have strong coping skills in place. The idea is to learn to apply the "brake" before using the "accelerator." This is especially true if you have both trauma problems and addiction, if either one is severe, or if you have any current serious problems such as homelessness, domestic violence, suicidal or violent impulses, or major mental illness. Addiction treatment programs emphasize present-focused models, too, with concepts such as "one day at a time," building recovery supports, and learning new coping skills to replace addictive behavior.

Do Past-Focused Work Carefully

Past-focused trauma counseling can be helpful if you're ready for it, you choose it, and you have a good counselor who's trained in it and knows how to pace it. But safeguards are needed. It's sometimes called "opening Pandora's box," as it moves into painful trauma memories and feelings that can be more intense than you're prepared to handle. The goal is balanced awareness about both the positive and negative potential of past-focused trauma counseling. If you have addiction as well as trauma problems, be sure your trauma counselor is knowledgeable about how that impacts the trauma work.

Sometimes past-focused trauma counseling goes awry even with well-intentioned counselors: too much pressure on you to do it; overselling ("It's the only way to recover"); not bringing you down from intense emotions by the end of the session; lack of procedures for what to do if you worsen; lack of attention to addictive behavior; doing it without enough support or time (e.g., as part of a drop-in group rather than regular counseling); not assessing your readiness carefully on the front end; or pushing you to keep going even if it's not helping.

Tell your counselor if you find yourself getting worse while doing past-focused trauma counseling. A good counselor will respond with empathy and help you come up with a clear plan for handling it.

✴ Explore . . . *Quiz: Two types of trauma counseling*

Here are the questions and answers to the quiz at the beginning of the chapter.

1. "Trauma counseling means you tell your trauma story (what happened) in detail."

   Under<u>False</u>. It will depend on what type of trauma counseling you choose to do. In present-focused trauma counseling you *don't* go into the details of your trauma story, but in past-focused trauma counseling you *do*. See the description of both types earlier in this chapter.

2. "You have to reduce your addictive behavior before you work on trauma."

   <u>False</u>. It's great if you can reduce your addictive behavior. But research shows that you don't have to do that before you work on trauma problems as long as you're doing present-focused trauma work (coping skills) or using a past-focused model that's adapted for people with addiction or provided in a context of strong addiction treatment.

3. "You need to tell your trauma story to recover fully."

<u>False</u>. Some people benefit and some don't. Many people recover without ever telling their story or focusing on the past. It's a choice, not a requirement.

4. "If you feel ready to tell your trauma story, you're ready."

<u>False</u>. Readiness is based on many factors, including being stable enough to do it safely, being with a counselor who's a good fit for you and trained to do it, and having strong coping skills. People often underestimate what the work will bring up or hold the naïve view that just spilling or "purging" their trauma story will resolve their problems.

5. "You can work on addiction and trauma at the same time."

<u>True</u>. Working on both at the same time can be done with a present-focused model or when a past-focused model adapted for addiction and trauma. The old approach was "First get your addiction under control and only then address trauma." The new approach is to work on both at the same time from the start of treatment. People with trauma and addiction problems prefer to work on both together, according to research.

6. "After you tell your trauma story, your addiction will go away."

<u>False</u>. Once you have an addiction, especially a serious one, it usually won't go away just through past-focused trauma counseling. You also need to work directly on the addiction. Some people find their addiction improves as they work on trauma (it's great if this happens), but this can't be assumed.

7. "The more intense the trauma counseling, the more you'll recover."

<u>False</u>. Many people have a gut sense this must be true ("no pain, no gain"), but research shows it's not. Generally, past-focused trauma counseling is more emotionally intense than present-focused counseling, but they do equally well in their results.

Much more research is needed on these topics, and the answers to the quiz may change as new studies emerge. Stay informed (see "Resources," Appendix B).

Sources: See References for further information on the points made in this chapter, especially Harned et al. (2014) and Najavits & Hien (2013).

✧ What type of trauma counseling appeals to you – present focused, past focused, or a combination?

✧ Have you tried different types of trauma therapy? What was most/least helpful for you?

RECOVERY VOICES
———◦◦◦———

Sasha – "It's incredibly freeing."

Sasha had severe PTSD and substance addiction. "It's so important to hear, 'There are two approaches. You have a choice, and you shouldn't feel pushed to do this or that.' I've talked to so many people at AA meetings who say, 'I'm not going back to therapy; they're going to make me talk about the trauma.' Almost every person I know with PTSD and addiction has said that. They're not going forward because they think they're going to have to retell it. My own experience is that I've done both types, present focused and past focused. I found that both were really helpful, indeed life-changing, but the past-focused has got to be done by someone competent who understands both PTSD and substance abuse. I had one therapist say, 'Well, you have to tell me what the trauma was; you're not going to get better if you don't. So tell me exactly what your brother did on that night.' And I told her, and she said, 'That's it? Well, according to the law, that wouldn't count as rape.' I shut down completely – it was like what my mom used to say to me, but now it was coming from a professional. That silenced me for a good 10 years; I mean, I just wasn't going to talk about it again and I kept drinking. Eventually I went back to therapy and found someone I liked. But I felt that I had gotten the message earlier that therapy was all about talking about my trauma, that that's what you're supposed to do, so I would just tell her stuff, and it was really triggering, and I got into a very bad place. I was in way over my head, and I was cutting and drinking. It snowballed very quickly, and she didn't know what to do. And then finally, thank goodness, I found a therapist who understood about both PTSD and addiction. We started with present focused and then moved on to past focused only once I was ready and only in small doses at a time, moving back and forth between them even then. So I think the main thing is, whatever type of trauma therapy you do, the therapist has to know how to guide people safely and has to understand about addiction. And it's important to emphasize that it's not necessary to tell your story; you may choose to or not, and you can still get better. It's incredibly freeing to know this."

34

What the wounded can give back

There is a wisdom that is woe; but there is a woe that is madness. And there is a Catskill eagle in some souls that can alike dive down into the blackest gorges, and soar out of them again and become invisible in the sunny spaces. And even if he for ever flies within the gorge, that gorge is in the mountains; so that even in his lowest swoop the mountain eagle is still higher than other birds upon the plain, even though they soar.

—HERMAN MELVILLE, 19th-century American writer

Recovery from trauma and addiction has no defined endpoint. A broken arm heals, and that's it; you return to life as it was before. But trauma and addiction recovery transform you. You're still you, but now incorporating a broader sense of yourself, your place in the world, and your connection to others. It's often described as tempered steel: wisdom from suffering has made you stronger and more resilient. This also means that you can inspire healing in others.

You may or may not decide to devote yourself to helping others. But whatever form your recovery takes, your emotional wounds can be transformed and create a ripple effect that impacts others. As the writer Pete Wilson puts it, "Yes, hurt people do hurt people. But what's equally true is that free people free people."

The concept of the *wounded healer* goes back to ancient times in the form of shamans, mystics, native healers, and medicine men. In the modern era, it's a central theme in the helping professions, with the term itself coined by Carl Jung, an early 20th-century psychiatrist. A study of counselors by Alison Barr in Scotland found that the majority reported entering the field based on a vision of helping that arose from their own suffering.

Emotional wounds from trauma and addiction can become a "privileged path" to transformative growth, both personal and societal, says Oliver Morgan in *Thoughts on the Interaction of Trauma, Addiction, and Spirituality.* Paul Levy provides a poignant description in his blog *Awaken in the Dream*:

> We step out of identifying ourselves in a personal way that's separate from others, and we step into, as if stepping into new clothes that are custom tailored just for us, a "novel" role which requires a more all-embracing and expansive identity. . . . We find ourselves instruments being moved by a greater, invisible hand, as if something vast, with more volume than our previously imagined selves is incarnating through us. To recognize this is to have a more open-ended and expansive sense of who we think we are, and who we imagine others are in relation to us.

The social purpose that survivors take on varies and may be formal or informal. Some survivors become 12-step sponsors or SMART Recovery facilitators. Some volunteer at rape crisis centers, homeless shelters, suicide hotlines, child abuse programs, domestic violence shelters, soup kitchens, or other places where the most traumatized addicted people come for help. Others become professional counselors, doctors, or religious leaders. For some, the mission is based on spiritual beliefs, while others are nonbelievers who view altruism itself as the guiding principle. Such life-mission work helps others and, equally important, reinforces one's own healing and continued growth. Indeed, many people are not aware that AA was founded on this principle. It wasn't designed as a support group for alcoholics just to come and *get* help but also one where they would help bring other alcoholics into recovery. It was conceived as bidirectional healing in which one's own and others' recovery were continually intertwined and mutually transformative.

The fields of trauma and addiction recovery arose as grassroots "bottom-up" social movements started by survivors themselves. AA was founded in the 1930s by Bill W. and Dr. Bob, two alcoholics, and became the most widespread addiction recovery model ever developed. Domestic violence and child abuse were recognized as serious issues primarily due to the women's movement of the 1960s. Testimony therapy arose in Chile in the 1970s as a response to communitywide torture and genocide. After the Vietnam War, military veterans created their own vet centers and "rap groups" to heal trauma when they felt it was not being addressed by the Veterans Administration system.

Both trauma and addiction represent, at their low point, a crisis of meaning: "Why did I have to go through this?" "How could people treat me this way?" "Am I defective?" "Am I alone in the world?" "Is there hope?" "Can people be good?" In the words of psychologists Oliver Morgan and Dusty Miller, "recovery from both addictions and trauma requires the restoration of hope . . . a sense of meaning, renewing relationships, and 'creating a reverence for life coupled with a sense of social purpose' are also critical."

But the wounded healer is double-edged – there's strength but also vulnerability. Healers can become burned out if they are so mission driven that they don't take care of their own needs for rest and time off. Seeing others with trauma and addiction can be triggering and may set off relapse. At times, healers may become "infected" by the problems of those they help. To truly help others means to also continue in your own recovery work.

✧ Would helping others interest you?

✧ How might helping others sustain your own recovery?

RECOVERY VOICES

Craig – "I've walked in their combat boots."

Craig served in the Army during the Vietnam War, was seriously wounded, and developed PTSD and alcohol abuse. After working on his own recovery, he became a social worker and eventually a team leader at a vet center. "There's a lot I can give back because I've done my own work. I've been in treatment for PTSD; I've been in AA for years and been sober for over 20 years; and I feel that because of these I can be a powerful healer. I have a lot of insight into veterans' problems and a lot of empathy. Having been in combat gives me a first-hand perspective. Being a wounded healer, being a Vietnam veteran, gives me credibility. I can say things to them that other treaters can't because I've walked in their combat boots. I use humor and pretty much say anything, and the guys will be cracking up; they get what I'm saying. If someone else tried it who hadn't been in combat or didn't have substance abuse, it just wouldn't work the same. They give me a lot of respect because I know the pain they're carrying.

"We wounded healers can also be great models for them, especially some of the young guys back from Iraq and Afghanistan. When they see me, a 70-year-old, they say 'Well, gee whiz, maybe I can reach that age too.' I remember when I first came home from Vietnam I never expected to live this long. It gives them hope – a sense that 'I can heal.' We watch them recover; we watch how these people who are lonely and helpless bond together into groups, re-creating their platoons in the military. I'm like the commanding officer, and they have all their buddies with them. Because of what I've experienced, I can be pretty useful to them. I talk about how I straightened out my life, my past.

"It plays a role in my own recovery too. Life for me became a wonderful ministry. It took on real meaning when I began to help others. It's about being honest, just like in the fourth step of AA, which talks about fearlessly searching for healing. I think that's one of the things as a treater that you really need – that honesty that's the exact opposite of the pathological symptoms. When you're having problems with substances or PTSD, you lie to yourself. So one of the first steps in healing is honesty. This book can help keep you from lying to yourself because you see yourself reflected in it: 'Oh yeah, that's me; and yeah, I do that too.' It can help them not to be afraid to expose who they are, to be vulnerable. It's done beautifully. When I read it, I said, wow, this is great stuff."

35

"We are all in the gutter, but some
of us are looking at the stars"

The title quote is from Oscar Wilde, a 19th-century Irish writer who suffered trauma and alcoholism.

Although this book ends, recovery continues. Recovery has many different meanings, but one of the most profound is that you learn to love who you *really* are. It may include loving some inner part of you that's deeper than your trauma and addiction (the timeless self that's always there beneath the surface); loving yourself for having survived and for who you can still become; loving that you still have life ahead. Charlotte Kasl, an addiction specialist, says, "People may give up addiction out of fear, but they heal out of love."

What does it look like? When you make a mistake, it means you find a way to forgive yourself, yet also try not to repeat the mistake next time. It means that when you have an urge to act on addictive impulses, you talk yourself through it in kind but firm ways. It means that when you start to "beat yourself up" you catch yourself and back off, recognizing that this is not a kind (or productive) way to change your behavior. It means you take care of your body and your environment. It means you give yourself praise when you do well and honest feedback when you don't do well. It means you allow yourself the full range of feelings, including anger, sadness, disappointment, hurt, and fear. It means you strive to respect yourself, recognizing that even with all that you've done and all that's happened to you, you have an essential core that's valuable. It means that even if others don't believe in you, you believe in you. It means that you try to overcome personality flaws through gentle encouragement. It means that when you get angry you listen to your feelings but don't act out on them. It means you become emotionally intimate with yourself, aware of the double-edged nature of your traits. It means you love yourself even though you may not love your weaknesses. It means you strive to see yourself and others clearly and act in accord with that knowledge. It means you hold yourself to a high standard.

This type of love is not narcissism – it's not believing that everything you do is great or that you deserve special treatment. It's about finding ways to encourage yourself so that you create a better life for yourself. It also doesn't require that someone else love you. Indeed, the more you grow love for yourself the more likely it is that others will be drawn to you and help support your best self.

These pursuits never end but keep reinforcing each other as you move forward into the future, simultaneous with all the realities of life, its ups and downs, hardships and pain, along the way.

☆ Explore . . . *And you?*

How far you have come in recovery? Where are you headed? Fill in the blanks for any questions below that you want to answer.

- I came to accept _____

  _____.

- I still have questions about _____

  _____.

- I want more _____

  _____.

- I am most proud of _____

  _____.

- I know I need to _____

  _____.

- Even if no one else gets it, what I know about myself is that _____

  _____.

- My recovery matters because _____
  _____.

- What I most want to strengthen is _____
  _____.

- What I most want to let go of is _____
  _____.

- The people who have made a real difference are _____
  _____.

- I have become hopeful about _____
  _____.

- I can further heal my trauma problems if I _____
  _____.

- I can further heal my addiction if I _____
  _____.

- One thing I need to do every day for recovery is _____
  _____.

- I find inspiration from _____
  _____.

- I believe I can be happy if I _____
  _____.

- What has helped me the most in this book is _____
  _____.

- My best advice to myself now is _____
  _____.

- My best coping skills are _____
  _____.

- My favorite quotes in this book are _____
  _____.

- I have become aware of _____
  _____.

- I have been able to grow in love toward _____
  _____.

✧ What can you do next to guide your recovery forward?

RECOVERY VOICES

David – "Recovery is full of new beginnings."

"Recovery is not something that's reached or achieved. Recovery is fluid, dynamic, diverse – recovery is life. Recovery is possible, but it is lived, not achieved like a goal that has an endpoint. It's full of new beginnings. An example of how far I've come: My wife Nora and I had to euthanize our greyhound Winston a little over a month ago. We got back from vacation with Winston (he accompanied us pretty much wherever we went), and when we got back he started getting sick. The pain I was able to experience, the vulnerability I was able to show in front of Nora and with Nora, the tears I was able to shed, the fear I was able to walk through the day we took him to the hospital – none of that would have been possible without recovery. To be able to show up and be with Winston and Nora and comfort him as he took his last breath and then to comfort Nora was beautiful – painful, but beautiful. Nora and I, having walked through that pain together, have a stronger relationship. On Friday, Nora and I are traveling north to adopt another greyhound named Jake, who we met last week. Life goes on – Nora and I love dogs, and Jake the greyhound needs a home and a lot of love. The depth of our suffering equals the potential depth of our joy, and in the transformation meaning is created. Trust grows brighter as night turns to day. You taught me that."

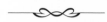

How others can help – family, friends, partners, sponsors, counselors

For, ultimately, and precisely in the deepest and most important matters, we are unspeakably alone, and many things must happen, many things must go right, a whole constellation of events must occur, for one human being to successfully advise or help another.

—Rainer Maria Rilke, 20th-century German writer

Do you want to help someone who has trauma or addiction problems?

This appendix offers help for the helper. You may be a partner, family member, friend, counselor, or 12-step sponsor, for example. This may be your first attempt at helping, or you may already be off to a good start and just want more guidance. Or you may be hitting a point of despair – the person keeps relapsing, shuts you out, or you're frightened about what may happen next such as suicide or violence.

Whatever your involvement, you can be incredibly important, even life-saving, to the person with trauma and addiction problems.

Kristin is 21 years old. She experimented with drugs in high school but became seriously addicted only after being sexually assaulted at a rave concert. "I'm amazed how my parents stood by me. They didn't know about the assault; I couldn't tell them; it made me nauseous just to think about it. But they saw I was sliding downhill: my grades were bad and I didn't care about anything anymore. They found pills in my bag and took me to treatment. That was how I first told someone about the assault, and it was the start of my recovery. My parents saw what I needed before I could see it."

Dilemmas

There are many dilemmas when helping someone with trauma and addiction problems:

- How to be present but not intrusive.
- What to do if the person is dragging you or your family down.
- How to cope with denial.
- Whether to let the person "hit bottom."
- When to give advice and when to step back.
- How to respond if the person gets angry or violent.
- What to do with your own feelings, especially if you have your own history of trauma or addiction.
- How to be kind without reinforcing destructive patterns.

Brock describes what it was like dealing with his severely alcoholic wife: "She lied all the time about her drinking. She resisted change. I was supportive and kind; I really loved her and wanted to believe her. I gave her every opportunity, but she blew it over and over. When I doubted her intentions, she was mortified and hurt that I would doubt her. She viewed me as the cause of her downfall. I felt completely alone, trapped. There was basically nothing I could do. I didn't want to abandon her, but after a while I did want to leave, to get away from it all. Things finally changed one night when I was really upset after she got fired from her job. I told her she had to move out. We agreed she'd go to rehab. The rehab wasn't a good experience for her, but it got her to AA. She had been to AA before, but it didn't 'take' back then. This time she found some cool people who were like the people she used to drink with. She wasn't even really friends with them, but it was just enough connection to get her truly involved in AA. It was finding people of her own 'tribe,' and it saved her life.

"When I look back on it, I had been addicted to an image of myself. I needed to see myself as a caring, generous person and someone who wasn't cowardly, that if I did the right things I could manage this. But I was completely enmeshed. The truth is that I was afraid of her, intimidated. I came to see that you can't control another person or shape the outcome no matter how hard you try. I really needed to let go of my illusions. I needed to be able to see the reality for what it was. The actual step of getting her to get help was so difficult for me. When I was able to accept the truth about her and about me, that's when I was finally able to say what I needed to say to her."

There are no easy answers, but the goal is to strive for what's most likely to succeed. You may have fine intentions but offer help that isn't useful or may even undermine recovery. Read on to explore how to invest your best efforts, marking any ideas you want to try.

The principles in this chapter apply to a broad range of people. The person you're trying to help may have just addiction, just trauma problems, or both. The person may have problem behavior (less severe) or full-blown conditions (more severe). The person may have additional life problems such as financial issues, homelessness, physical illness, or legal problems. He or she may have one addiction such as substance abuse or multiple ones such as addiction to gambling, sex, pornography, or shopping/spending. For more about these issues, see "It's medical – you're not crazy, lazy, or bad" (Chapter 4).

If you're reading this book for your own recovery . . .

You can give this chapter to someone in your life. But be sure it's a *safe* person – someone who:

- Is not currently harming you.
- Is not currently struggling with a major addiction.
- Is reasonably stable.
- Has your best interests at heart.

If no one in your life is safe, you can still get help from a counselor, 12-step sponsor, or other formal helper.

You can also read this chapter for yourself to learn more about how others can support your recovery.

A Starting Point: Two Questions for the Helper

Reflect on the two questions that follow. No matter what your answers are, you can read the rest of this chapter and explore ways to help. But if you say "no" to one or both questions, be cautious. A key principle of helping is *first, do no harm*. This means that it's sometimes better to step back and do nothing than to jump in and do something that may cause harm. Your honest self-awareness is the starting point.

Question 1: Are you in a good enough place in your own life to help someone else?

There's a saying that "you can't teach someone what you don't already know." You need to be at least one step ahead of – more stable than – the person you're trying to help. If you're in recovery yourself, that's fine if it's sustained, typically for a year or more. If you have major current addiction, trauma problems, mental illness, or major stress in your own life such as divorce or job loss, you likely need to take care of yourself first. Your living example of stability is more powerful than words: show it, don't just say it. If you need to help yourself first, let the person know that. You can still offer practical help such as making phone calls or providing transportation, rather than trying to intervene on an emotional level.

Question 2: Do you have a good enough relationship with the person you're trying to help?

Your relationship needs to be strong enough for the person to trust your motives and really hear you at least some of the time. If there's too much fighting, distancing, or distrust, you may not be able to help and may cause further harm. The person may act out and do the opposite of what you say just to spite you. The person may get into power struggles to prove you wrong ("I don't need anyone's help"). Or there may be positive words but no action ("Sure, I'll go to AA, but not this week").

Your relationship is like flooring that needs to be sturdy enough to "walk" with the person without either of you falling through. This means there's positive energy in the relationship. You value each other. You care about the person's welfare. You're open with each other. You can respectfully disagree. You can resolve conflicts without physical or emotional violence.

Important changes often happen because of a good relationship. Maybe you can be that presence.

If you're a professional helper, ask your client to fill out the Helping Alliance Questionnaire in "Find a good counselor" (Chapter 32). A strong alliance is associated with greater treatment success.

How to Help

Learn All You Can about Trauma and Addiction

The more you learn about trauma and addiction, the stronger your help will be. You may be surprised to hear, for example, that . . .

- There's no known addictive personality.
- People can recover from trauma without telling the painful, detailed story of it.
- People can recover from addiction even if they start out unwilling or unmotivated to give it up.
- Working on trauma and addiction *at the same time* is recommended rather than addiction first, then trauma.
- Twelve-step groups such as Alcoholics Anonymous can be super helpful but aren't required for addiction recovery.
- The longer a person stays in addiction treatment, the better the results.
- Early help is best; don't wait for the person to "hit bottom."
- Both addiction and trauma problems run in families and have a genetic basis.
- There are many ways to succeed at recovery: "Many roads, one journey."
- Trauma can lead to addiction, but addiction can lead to trauma too.

Read as much as you can of this book. See "Resources" (Appendix B) for further ways to learn. And try taking the quiz in Appendix D.

Try to Really Understand How Hard It Is for the Person

It's important to get how difficult it may be for the person to change. If you haven't had addiction or trauma problems, it may seem much easier than it is. You may be able to stop after one drink or gamble $50 and leave the casino. You may have survived trauma and moved on. But the person you're helping may be different – lost, confused, unable to take action or make decisions.

Linda was abused as a child. "The world out there doesn't have a clue. You feel alone, isolated, weird, crazy sometimes. He used to tell me that the reason he was molesting me was that he loved me. And I had every reason to believe him because I did adore him. It messed with my head – about what is real and what isn't real." Later in life she couldn't figure out who to trust. She had difficulty making decisions and thinking straight because she constantly doubted herself. Teachers at school and work supervisors, unaware of her trauma history, assumed she just wasn't smart or wasn't trying hard enough.

—Adapted from the video *Counting the Cost: The Lasting Impact of Childhood Trauma*

See the section "What Can Help, What Can Harm" below through page 238 for examples of what it sounds like to respond with understanding (and lack of understanding).

Do the Exercises in This Book as If You're the Other Person

Try the exercises in this book as an imagination experiment that can deepen your awareness of what the person is going through. In the trauma field, there's a helpful phrase: "See the world through the lens of trauma." Difficult behavior makes more sense if it's understood in light of trauma. For example, someone who survived war may view others as the enemy; someone who was neglected as a child may appear "entitled" and "demanding." You can also look through the lens of addiction. A person may minimize addiction out of shame or lie about it to save face; when people feel out of control, it makes sense that they try to hide it. The person may look tough but be fragile inside.

What Can Help, What Can Harm

Circle anything below that you want to work on.

What can *help*	What it sounds like
Listening without judgment	"I want to hear what you're going through. I'll just listen."
Encouragement	"I believe in you"; "There really is hope"; "Others have gotten better, and so can you."
Building trust slowly	"It may take a while for us to trust each other."
Offering options rather than "one right way"	"Let's brainstorm some options, and you can pick what you prefer."

What can *help*	What it sounds like
Validation	"You have every right to your feelings"; "It makes sense that you feel that way."
Openness	"I want to know what's really going on."
Questions	"What would help the most right now?"; "How can I support you?"
Practical support	"Call me any time, day or night"; "I can help you find a counselor if you want."
Moral support	"No child ever deserves that"; "No matter what you wore, he didn't have the right to attack you."
Focusing on the present	"Let's figure out what can help you now."
Empathy	"I hear the sadness in your voice."
Noticing strengths	"I'm so impressed by your resilience"; "You're a survivor."
Reaching out	"I'm calling to check in and see how you're doing."

What can *harm*	What it sounds like
Invalidating the person's perspective	"Those are just excuses"; "Stop saying that."
Being unrealistic	"Just don't drink"; "You'll feel better soon."
Negating trauma	"Forget about it; it's over"; "You're young enough – just have another child."
Negating addiction	"Everyone drinks"; "You don't look like an addict."
Insisting that what worked for you will work for them	"Just go to AA; that's what I did."

What can *harm*	What it sounds like
Making assumptions	"You need to tell your story"; "You have to forgive the person who hurt you."
False reassurance	"Everything happens for a reason"; "Time heals all wounds."
Moralizing	"Using drugs is wrong"; "You shouldn't have dressed that way."
Asking for upsetting details	"Tell me exactly what happened during the trauma."
Focusing on the past	"It all started when you were a kid . . ."; "Your parents should have done more."
Breaking promises	"I meant to visit you in the hospital, but I got too busy."
Accusing	"I'll bet you drank again"; "Stop being such a victim."
Demanding information	"Tell me who in your family abused you."

Notice what these examples convey. You are most helpful when . . .

- You're the listener more than the talker.
- You take the problems seriously.
- You get how hard it feels for the person.
- You respect the person's boundaries.
- You strive to build genuine trust.
- You offer but don't impose your solutions.
- You create an atmosphere of hope.
- You listen for *feelings* the person is expressing.
- You understand that you can validate feelings without having to agree with the other person's point of view.
- You don't delve into upsetting material unless it's a counseling context and mutually agreed upon.

Balance Love and Limits

A common response to people with addiction and trauma problems is to be either *too nice* or *too harsh*. You may also find yourself bouncing between these.

Too nice. You may believe that "love cures all." Your support can be extremely helpful, but if taken too far it can undermine the person's recovery. *Enabling* is an addiction term that refers to making excuses for the person's behavior, which perpetuates the addiction. Enabling means not setting reasonable boundaries, and looking the other way, pretending things are better than they really are. Enabling also occurs in response to trauma, such as tolerating someone physically hurting you ("Deep down, he's just in a lot of pain"). Being too nice can also wear you out. Helpers who offer love without limits become exhausted and resentful, diminishing their capacity to help. So both for your sake and for the other person, be kind but not at the expense of being real.

Too harsh. This means being unsympathetic, too confrontational, and over-controlling. You may use phrases such as "zero tolerance," "my way or the highway," "three strikes and you're out," and other all-or-none positions. This strict stance is usually too tough and can lead people to fail even when they are genuinely trying to succeed. It may drive them to the streets or to unsafe people out of a desperate desire for support. Also, people with a trauma history may perceive harshness as neglect or abuse even if you don't mean it that way. Frank is a man with opiate addiction who was emotionally abused by his father. He says, "I already hate myself more than you can ever hate me. When you talk to me like you're mad at me, it doesn't make me change; it just makes me want to hide from you."

Balance. The goal is to *balance* love and limits. Give support, but be clear on your boundaries. Offer help, but take care of yourself too. Be kind, but also offer honest feedback. Enforce consequences that are fair but not so harsh that they set the person up to fail. This is where it's crucial to understand trauma as well as addiction. In classic addiction-only care having the person "hit bottom" or staging an intervention to gather everyone together to confront the addict sometimes works as a last-ditch effort to get the person to face consequences and finally make changes. But when someone has trauma problems or other major mental health issues, those strategies often backfire because the emotional problems are not addressed. The "bottom" keeps dropping, and the person may end up cutting off all contact or just giving up altogether. Even if the person desperately wants to do the right thing, the emotional problems can get in the way. There are medications and counseling for emotional problems that can help the person succeed in addiction recovery. The addiction field has come a long way since the 1935 founding of AA when such medications and counseling were not available. There are even medications that curb substance cravings. Research shows that providing all possible treatment for as long as possible is the best path to successful recovery. New methods are continually evolving, so even if something didn't work before, try reaching out again to find new options that may be available.

The goal is balance rather than extremes. Instead of "If you don't go to AA, I'll throw you out of the house," try setting up a plan, perhaps with a counselor's help, to reinforce clear steps that set up rewards for successes and a carefully planned set of consequences. The consequences need to be strong enough to matter but not so strong that they'll break the person. If you have no consequences – no limits or requirements – you may reinforce the person's problems and build up your own resentments. The consequences will depend on who you are, who the other person is, what your relationship is, your power in the person's life, how motivated the person is, and how serious the problems are. If needed, get guidance from others to come up with a plan. You may also need to experiment a lot to find solutions that work. If the person you're trying to help has a history of suicide or violence toward others, get professional help to figure out what to do. Don't put yourself or others in danger. And if you do decide to stage an intervention, explore more gentle versions that have been developed in recent years rather than the harsh old-school approach.

Avoid Harsh Confrontation

Harsh confrontation used to be the hallmark of addiction treatment: "Break 'em down to build 'em up." To challenge the denial that's often part of severe addiction, addiction programs used methods such as the "hot seat," "emotional surgery," the "haircut," and forcing people to wear humiliating signs or endure punishments like cleaning toilets. But in the past several decades, research has shown that support helps more than confrontation. A study done more than 20 years ago by psychologist Bill Miller and colleagues found that the more counselors confronted problem drinkers about their drinking the more the clients drank. (See "Resources," Appendix B, for a fascinating article by Miller and White describing the history of harsh confrontation models and the lack of positive evidence for them.) Such methods are still used in some programs, but current best practices in addiction treatment emphasize collaboration, holding to limits in kind ways, and offering realistic encouragement. This is true for addiction alone and all the more important in the context of major vulnerabilities such as trauma, homelessness, domestic violence, head injury, serious physical health problems, or mental illness.

Empower the Person

Strive to empower the person you're helping. Offer choices ("What would you like to talk about?"); ask permission ("Can we talk more about that?"); seek feedback ("Was this helpful to you?"); and encourage the person to notice what feels right ("Would it help to try counseling?"). Such collaborative approaches are especially important for people with addiction and trauma problems. The nature of both is to feel powerless. Trauma is rooted in lack of power; people don't choose to be traumatized. And many traumas represent major abuse of power such as torture, child abuse, and domestic violence. Addiction, too, means people feel powerless to change their own behavior. But empowerment doesn't mean letting them "walk all over you" or agreeing with everything they say. Equally important is accountability – conveying that they're responsible for acting in safe, respectful, healthy ways.

Be Honest – What Are You Feeling?

You may have many positive feelings toward the person – caring, love, protective-ness. But it's also common to want to feel more positive than you really do. You may feel guilty about being angry or tired of the person's problems. You may think that because the person suffered trauma you need to be a "saint," always sympathetic. You may believe you shouldn't doubt or mistrust the person even though you keep getting lied to. Know that it's normal to have mixed feelings. You don't have to express your feelings out loud, but you do need to honestly own them within yourself. Your feel-ings are like a thermometer that tells you the temperature. They help you "dress for the weather" – to prepare for how you'll respond to the person in an authentic way. Observe what comes up in your body and your heart. Common feelings when deal-ing with someone with serious trauma and addiction problems include the following:

- Worn out; you've given all you can.
- Sadness at what the person has suffered.
- Heartbroken about who the person has become.
- Furious about being betrayed or having promises broken.
- Afraid to say anything; it's like "walking on eggshells."
- Moral outrage if you see the person hurt others.
- Resentful about how much you've had to sacrifice.
- Helpless if the person shuts you out.
- Unsafe, not sure what the person may do next.

- Envious of the attention the person gets.
- Confused; you want to help but don't know how.
- Guilty about what you did or didn't do.
- Angry that the person is dragging you down.
- Triggered into your own trauma or addiction reactions.
- Not caring anymore.

Never Underestimate the Power of Addiction

When severe, addiction is like a set of iron claws that takes hold and won't let go. You're never, ever stronger than those claws. It's sad, but at its worst, addiction is more important than family, a job, children, and right or wrong. If you say to yourself, "I just need to love this person more," you may be living an illusion just like the addicted person does. The best approach is to respond to the person based on behavior you can see and verify. Credit card statements reveal gambling or spending problems. Empty pill bottles reveal drug abuse. Actively look for clues and information. The person may be trying to convince everyone that there's progress or a new path, but you need to see actions, not just words. If you find evidence of addictive behavior, consider how you'll respond – not lashing out but taking the *love and limits* approach described earlier. People with addiction can recover, but it requires great effort on their part. You can help, but you can't do it for them.

Never Underestimate the Power of Trauma

Trauma problems can overwhelm a person far longer and stronger than anyone expects. Try to get the person as much professional support as you can if problems persist. Also be aware that trauma can have a ripple effect: families, friends, and helpers may become "contaminated" by the person's intense feelings, sometimes developing trauma-related problems that mirror those of the traumatized person. You may have nightmares about the person's trauma. You may want to lash out against a trauma perpetrator. This is called *vicarious trauma, PTSD by contact,* or *secondary PTSD.* Take care of yourself as well as the other person.

Be Willing to Have the Person Dislike You

People with severe trauma and addiction problems may act destructively yet be only partially aware of what they're doing due to intoxication, numbness, or dissociation (the latter is a sort of "spacing out" that occurs in highly traumatized people). They may have good intentions that fall away as soon as they're triggered into old patterns. They may be so despairing that they don't care what happens. Emotionally, they may be like children at times, without the maturity to take care of themselves. As a helper, your role is best described as being like a kind but firm parent. You're in touch with reality and doing all you can to keep the person safe. You're the one who sometimes has to say what's hard to say and do what's hard to do. You may have to call the person's doctor to reveal the extent of the addiction. You may have to take action to protect a child who's being neglected or abused. The person may feel bitter resentment in the moment. If you know you're doing what's right, take comfort in that; later, the person may come to appreciate that you did what had to be done. Whatever the tough moments are, offer as much compassion as possible to the person – no putdowns or name-calling.

Go to a Self-Help Meeting

Self-help groups are widely available for addiction but not for trauma problems (although you can try searching online for trauma self-help groups). Thus the focus here will be addiction self-help groups. First and most important, try Al-Anon (*www. al-anon.org*), which offers free local support groups for anyone whose life is affected by a person with addiction. Friends and family can attend as well as counselors and other professionals. You can share experiences and explore how to respond to the addicted person. You can also attend an open 12-step meeting. You don't have be addicted yourself, and you don't have to speak. Listening to people talk about their addiction and recovery can be eye-opening. Meetings can also be very moving as people share their "experience, strength, and hope" (a well-known AA phrase). There are many different 12-step groups such as Alcoholics Anonymous, Cocaine Anonymous, Narcotics Anonymous, Workaholics Anonymous, Overeaters Anonymous, Sexaholics Anonymous, and Gamblers Anonymous. Depending on where you live, there may also be SMART Recovery, Rational Recovery, Women for Sobriety, and other alternatives to 12-step meetings. See "Resources" (Appendix B) for how to locate self-help groups.

Have an Emergency Plan

Scary moments arise when the person becomes agitated, suicidal, violent, or a danger to children. Don't try to handle these situations alone. Addiction can turn people into someone they're not, and the situation can become volatile when mixed with trauma problems. People are more likely to commit suicide or violence when they're intoxicated, for example. Severe PTSD can lead people to wake up from a nightmare choking their partner. Yet most people with trauma and addiction never physically hurt themselves or others. If they do become violent, it's much more often aimed at themselves rather than others. So don't fall into unhealthy fear of the person, which can create distance when the person most needs your help. But do prepare for possible emergencies just in case. Know where your nearest emergency room is, what hotline numbers are available, and whether the person has any mental health providers you can get in touch with if needed. See "Resources" (Appendix B) for options, including a suicide phone app. If you need help figuring out an emergency plan, you may benefit from a session with a local social worker, psychiatrist, or other mental health professional. If the person becomes a threat to self or others, get immediate help; never allow a dangerous situation to continue.

Honor Your Own History

Trauma and addiction are common, and you may have a history of one or both. Most people survive a trauma in their lifetime. And addiction is widespread. (If you're unsure whether you've had trauma or addiction, see "Resources," Appendix B, for how to locate free, brief, online anonymous screening tests.) To *honor your history* means recognizing strengths that arose from your difficult experiences. But it also means you may have unfinished business that can get in the way of helping someone else. You may become easily triggered and upset with the person you're trying to help. You may fall into some of the harmful messages described earlier in this chapter. You may avoid facing what's really going on.

"Beth's parents were alcoholic. As a child, she did everything possible to look good or be good. The violence and punishment were so great in her family that she went to any extent to avoid conflict. The extra efforts at school, her extracurricular activities, and her jobs served many purposes. She was away from home as much as possible, she did not get into trouble, and she received attention for doing well. Although competent, Beth felt inadequate most of the time. She believed she had to prove herself over and over. . . . In treatment, Beth realized that her history with [her husband, an alcoholic and sex addict] revealed a consistent process in which she sacrificed her own identity – giving up a part of herself in order to stay in the relationship. This process included a range of strategies:

- Disregarding her own intentions
- Overlooking behavior that hurt her deeply
- Covering up behavior that she despised
- Appearing cheerful when she was hurting
- Avoiding conflict to keep up appearances
- Allowing herself to be disrespected repeatedly
- Allowing her own standards to be compromised
- Faulting herself for the family's problems
- Believing she had no options

Everything Beth did was similar to what she had done to survive as a child in an alcoholic family.
—From *Out of the Shadows: Understanding Sexual Addiction,* by Patrick Carnes

---

Get yourself help if needed. The more you heal, the more you can truly help others.

Offer Practical Support

Practical support can take many forms, such as:

- Guiding the person to a counselor, support groups, or other formal help.
- Checking in to see how the person is doing.
- Creating a clear written plan for what to do in case of emergency.
- Transporting the person to treatment.
- Offering books and online resources.
- Helping with child care.

Be Prepared for Intense Dynamics

The more complex the person's history of trauma and addiction, the more likely you are to encounter challenging dynamics. Such patterns typically arise from painful feelings the person doesn't know how to manage. Strive for compassion while also responding effectively, which may include limit setting, skill building, and getting help for the person and for yourself. Difficult dynamics include:

- *"Walking into danger."* The person lacks self-protection and keeps getting involved with harmful people and dangerous situations.

- *Poor self-care.* The person doesn't keep up with basics such as hygiene and nutrition.

- *Lashing out.* The person pushes others away, blows up in anger, or rejects help.

- *Failure of empathy.* The person can't take another person's perspective; ignores obvious needs of his/her own children; may justify criminal behavior.

- *Regression.* The person becomes dependent and childlike.

- *Distrust.* The person feels that no one can be trusted; you're shut out.

- *Destructive behavior.* The person acts recklessly such as driving drunk; engages in self-injury such as cutting; or harms others (assault, emotional abuse).

- *Too much or too little responsibility. Too much* means harsh self-blame; *too little* means blaming everyone else for everything.

- *Continual crisis.* The person is in constant havoc: fired from jobs, explosive relationship breakups. Such people may seem addicted to "drama," but it's the chaos and pain of their internal world reflected in the outside world.

Keep Seeing the Good in the Person

Strive to hang on to what you like and admire about the person. The more extreme the person becomes, the more extreme your reactions may become. You may lose a sense of balance: being able to love the person even though some aspects are not so lovable. You may become blind to what's good.

Remember That Helping Can Be Deeply Rewarding

Helping can bring real gratification. For example, research shows that counselors who treat people with addiction and trauma problems report significantly more positives than negatives in the work. Watching recovery happen is sometimes described in spiritual terms as grace unfolding. Recovery does happen, often in unexpected ways for unexpected people.

RECOVERY VOICES

---∽∾⌇---

Margo – "It's a stronger, more real love now."

Margo's partner, Joe, became addicted to painkillers after a car accident left him with physical injuries as well as PTSD. "This chapter brings back a lot of what I went through with Joe. There's wisdom here that I wish I'd known then. I felt paralyzed for a long time not knowing what to do. The way I see it, Joe was terrified of stopping the addiction and used every tool, every weapon in his arsenal, conscious or unconscious, to keep the addiction going. He kept saying he was getting things under control, but I kept finding things like empty pill bottles and voicemails from different doctors who were prescribing the same painkillers.

"My father had been an alcoholic and died of cirrhosis. I swore I'd never get involved with an addict. I couldn't live that life again – the ups and downs, broken promises, watching him die of addiction and not being able to stop it. So when Joe developed his addiction I shut down. We had been together for 15 years by then, and I couldn't imagine life without him; I loved him more than anything. But I got triggered into my own past about my dad and felt doomed. I waited too long to act, and that didn't help either of us. I kept treading water, getting more and more depressed. I'm educated and think of myself as competent, but I sort of gave up inside. I didn't want to get into the crazy arguments I saw between my parents when I was growing up, trying to persuade the person to stop. It felt like there were no real options other than staying in this quagmire or leaving him, which broke my heart.

"What finally happened was that I became so depressed that I saw a psychiatrist and got on an antidepressant. That helped some, but the biggest thing was that he referred me to a social worker for counseling. She pieced together that Joe probably had PTSD, not just addiction. Everyone, including me, was so focused on Joe's physical injuries and the addiction that his PTSD went unnoticed. The social worker got me to see it and referred Joe to PTSD treatment. I was relieved to see that this didn't have to be a repeat of what I went through with my dad.

"I know I didn't save Joe – with addiction, people have to save themselves. But I related to him in new ways once I understood the PTSD. And he was able to get more on board with recovery once he saw how it connected to his addiction. It was a mix of my getting educated and his responding. It's kismet or luck; it might happen or not that the person responds. You have to do your best and allow for what unfolds. At the time, it felt miserable. I had to admit that I was scared of being alone, that nothing would work, and that I'd have to walk out on him for good.

"When I look back, it's the closest thing I've seen in my life to a miracle – that someone actually changed. In life, you bet on the past and it seems like no one really changes. Change is a hard thing, an unpredictable thing, but I've seen it happen. My dad didn't, but Joe did. I'm proud of him; I give him a lot of credit for what he did. And I feel like I did the right thing for myself. I walked a tight-rope, navigated a maze, and came out with more compassion toward both of us. I found options other than shutting down depressed or leaving in a furious rage. He's been off drugs for 5 years now and went back to work. He gets it now about being responsible for his feelings – not thrilled about it every day; it kinda sucks sometimes, dealing with what comes up rather than escaping through drugs. And he's still difficult at times. It's hard for him if you disagree with him; he doesn't take it well. We still have problems between us to deal with. But it's awe-some to see who he's become and how we can talk about things now. It's a stron-ger, more real love, not avoiding conflicts and hiding from the tough stuff, and that's more powerful than anything."

KEY POINTS FOR HELPERS

- Start by noticing whether you're in a good-enough place in your own life and have a good-enough relationship with the person you're trying to help.

- *Understanding* is the cornerstone of help; be aware of messages that help versus those that harm.

- Try completing the exercises in this book as if you were the person you're try-ing to help; see the world through that person's eyes.

- Be honest about your full range of feelings.

- Get help for your own trauma and/or addiction problems if needed.

- Above all, *balance love and limits*.

- Don't use harsh confrontation; the old "break 'em down to build 'em up" is no longer recommended.

- Never underestimate the power of addiction or of major trauma problems.

- Try Al-Alon to obtain support for you as a helper and sit in on a 12-step group such as Alcoholics Anonymous to hear moving stories about the "experience, strength, and hope" that addicted people share.

- Provide practical as well as emotional assistance.

- Create an emergency plan and get help to manage serious situations such as violence or suicide.

- Keep learning; there are many surprises about trauma and addiction recovery.

- Remember what you love about the person.

APPENDIX B

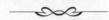

Resources

These resources are free and are from reputable government or nonprofit organizations. The list includes phone apps, hotlines, information, support, referral to treatment, and assessment tools. Each section also offers online search terms to help you find more. For books, see References.

Note: Any resource below that has a hotline or helpline is indicated with an asterisk (*).

Trauma/PTSD

Apps

Try free apps such as *Circle of 6, PTSD Coach, Mindshift,* and *T2 Mood Tracker.*

Online Search Terms

For trauma treatment or support, search "help for trauma," "trauma survivors support group," "PTSD support," and "PTSD treatment." For tools to help identify whether you have trauma problems, search "free trauma screening" and "free PTSD screening."

Organizations

Adverse Childhood Experiences Study
This website provides information on how child abuse and neglect contribute to problems later in life, including medical illness; as well as free online screening.
www.acestudy.org

Anxiety and Depression Association of America

This website offers online screening for PTSD, a free brochure, and other information.

www.adaa.org/screening-posttraumatic-stress-disorder-ptsd

Behavioral Health Treatment Locator

The Substance Abuse and Mental Health Services Administration offers this online tool to help you search for local treatment programs.

https://findtreatment.samhsa.gov

National Alliance on Mental Illness

This website provides support and referral for mental illness, including PTSD.

www.nami.org

National Centers for PTSD

This Veterans Affairs website provides resources relevant to military veterans and PTSD.

www.ptsd.va.gov

National Child Traumatic Stress Network

This website offers information to help improve care for children, adolescents, and families who have suffered trauma.

www.nctsn.org

*National Disaster Distress Helpline

The Substance Abuse and Mental Health Services Administration provides this crisis support helpline to help communities after disasters such as hurricanes, mass violence, floods, earthquakes, or wildfires.

Toll-free: 800-985-5990

www.samhsa.gov/find-help/disaster-distress-helpline

*National Domestic Violence Hotline

Domestic violence victims can access this free hotline 24/7.

Toll-free: 800-799-7233

www.thehotline.org

National Institute of Mental Health

This website provides information on trauma, PTSD, and other mental health issues.

www.nimh.nih.gov/health/topics/post-traumatic-stress-disorder-ptsd/index.shtml

National Resource Center on Domestic Violence
This website offers information on domestic violence prevention and treatment.
www.nrcdv.org

Addiction/Substance Abuse

Apps

Free apps are available to count drinks (e.g., *AlcoDroid*), to monitor gambling cravings (e.g., *MYGU*), and to provide recovery education. Search "free addiction help apps."

Online Search Terms

For treatment or support, search "addiction help," "support groups for addiction" (or "alcohol," etc.). For tools to help identify whether you have an addiction problem, search "free addiction screening tools" (also "free alcohol screening tool," "drug screening tool," "gambling screening tool," etc.).

Organizations

Twelve-step addiction self-help groups
Free local and telephone support groups that use the 12-step program.
For alcohol (*www.aa.org*); gambling (*www.gamblersanonymous.org*), overeating (*www.oa.org*), overspending (*www.debtorsanonymous.org*), sex addiction (*www.sa.org*), cocaine (*www.ca.org*), narcotics (*www.na.org*), nicotine (*www.nicotine-anonymous.org*), and for family members (*www.al-anon.org*). An online search can yield additional 12-step groups.

Harm Reduction Coalition
This website provides information on preventing overdoses and reducing stigma for drug users.
www.harmreduction.org

National Council on Alcoholism and Drug Dependence
Information and referrals for people with substance abuse problems and their families.
www.ncadd.org

*National Helpline
This 24/7 helpline by the Substance Abuse and Mental Health Services Administration provides information and referral to treatment for substance abuse and mental illness.
Toll-free: 800-662-HELP
www.samhsa.gov/find-help/national-helpline

National Institute on Alcohol Abuse and Alcoholism

This website provides information on alcohol abuse.

www.niaaa.nih.gov

National Institute on Drug Abuse

This website offers information on drug abuse.

www.nida.nih.gov

Rethinking Drinking

This website by the National Institute on Alcohol Abuse and Alcoholism provides interactive tools that can help you identify whether you have an alcohol problem, monitor your alcohol use (calories, cost, etc.), and get treatment referrals.

http://rethinkingdrinking.niaaa.nih.gov

SMART Recovery

SMART Recovery is a self-help organization that offers an alternative to AA, focusing on a skill-building, secular (non-spiritual) approach. The website has listings of free local and online groups.

www.smartrecovery.org

Vet Change

Vet Change provides online self-help tools for military veterans about PTSD and substance abuse.

www.vetchange.org

Suicide Prevention

Apps

There are many free apps such as *MY3, A Friend Asks, Stay Alive,* and *Operation Reach Out.* Search for additional apps with the term "free suicide prevention apps."

Online Search Terms

Try terms such as "suicide prevention," "help for suicidal person," and "suicidal thoughts."

Organizations

American Foundation for Suicide Prevention

This website offers education and advocacy to prevent suicide.

www.afsp.org

*National Suicide Prevention Lifeline
This 24/7 hotline is an immediate resource for people who feel suicidal.
Toll free: 800-273-TALK
www.suicidepreventionlifeline.org

HIV/AIDS

Resources for HIV/AIDS are listed here because both trauma and some addictions, such as substance abuse, increase the risk for HIV/AIDs.

Online Search Terms

Search "HIV help," "HIV prevention," "AIDS treatment" (etc.).

Organizations

*Centers for Disease Control and Prevention
This website has a toll-free hotline for locating HIV and STD testing.
800-CDC-INFO
https://gettested.cdc.gov

*Health Resources and Services Administration: HIV/AIDS Programs
This website provides a list of each state's HIV/AIDS toll-free hotline.
http://hab.hrsa.gov/gethelp/statehotlines.html

National Library of Medicine
This website offers HIV/AIDS information resources.
http://sis.nlm.nih.gov/hiv

Prevention Resources for People Living with AIDS
This website offers information to help prevent transmission of HIV.
www.cdc.gov/actagainstaids/campaigns/hivtreatmentworks/resources

U.S. Department of Health and Human Services
This website provides a free online tool to locate local HIV testing, as well as general HIV information.
www.hiv.gov

Additional Medical Information

You can search the world's medical literature for free to learn about any physical or mental health issue.

For example, if you want information on medications for PTSD, use either of the resources below and type in "medication and PTSD." It will pull up a description of each article that uses those terms. You can use the term "review" to find summary articles (e.g., "review and medication and PTSD").

The medical literature is written in technical language for professionals. See the resources earlier in this appendix for easier-to-read information.

Google Scholar

This resource provides free online access to the medical literature.
https://scholar.google.com

Pubmed

PubMed offers free online access to summaries of medical articles from the U.S. National Library of Medicine; the site's tutorials offer step-by-step search instructions.
www.ncbi.nlm.nih.gov/pubmed

~∞~

Excessive Behavior Scale

PART A: TYPES OF EXCESSIVE BEHAVIORS

Almost any behavior can become a problem *if you engage in it too much.*

For example, some people have problems from excessive gambling, eating, sex, shopping, work, exercise, Internet use, pornography, hair-pulling, skin-picking, tanning, or tattooing.

You may notice an excessive behavior in yourself based on any or all of the following:

- Spending too much time on it
- A feeling that you can't stop
- The toll it takes on your life – money problems, family or social problems (people complaining about the behavior), or medical or legal problems
- Control issues: sometimes it makes you feel more in control but at other times as if you've lost control
- The compulsion to do it
- The pleasure you take in it

On the next pages, circle each behavior that *may have been excessive for you for at least one month in the past year.* *You do not have to be certain about it.* You can base it on what you notice about yourself or what others say about you. Be honest, even if you are embarrassed or unsure. This survey is totally *confidential.*

	Excessive for at least 1 month in the past year?
a. Gambling (lottery, keno, sports betting, poker, etc.)	Yes / Maybe / No
b. Alcohol or drugs (cocaine, marijuana, heroin, oxycodone, etc.) List which (if more than one, pick the worst one):	Yes / Maybe / No
c. Working	Yes / Maybe / No
d. A leisure activity (such as TV, watching sports, a hobby such as fishing, going to psychics, fantasy football, etc.) List which:	Yes / Maybe / No
e. Exercising or doing a sport (such as running or baseball)	Yes / Maybe / No
f. Food (too much or too little, i.e., bingeing or restricting) List which:	Yes / Maybe / No
g. Use of electronics (texting, email, web surfing, computer games) List which:	Yes / Maybe / No
h. Body improvement (such as tattooing, plastic surgery, tanning) List which:	Yes / Maybe / No
i. A nervous habit (such as hair pulling, skin picking, chewing ice, etc.) List which:	Yes / Maybe / No

	Excessive for at least 1 month in the past year?
j. **Sex-related activities** (such as pornography, sex, sexual fetishes) List which:	Yes / Maybe / No
k. **"Too loose" with money** (such as shopping or overspending) List which:	Yes / Maybe / No
l. **"Too tight" with money** (such as acquiring or hoarding money) List which:	Yes / Maybe / No
m. **Hurting self or others physically** (cutting, burning, hitting, etc.) List whether self or others: List which type of behavior:	Yes / Maybe / No
n. **Criminal activity** (such as stealing, setting fires, etc.) List which:	Yes / Maybe / No
o. **Relationships** ("co-dependency" or "love addiction") List which:	Yes / Maybe / No
p. **A specific emotion** (anger or sadness, etc.) List which:	Yes / Maybe / No
q. **Others?** List which:	Yes / Maybe / No

PART B: SCREENING QUESTIONS

Step 1: Take the *first* excessive behavior that you checked off as Yes or Maybe in Part A and answer the grid of eight questions below in relation to that behavior.

For example, if you checked off Yes or Maybe to *gambling,* answer each of the eight questions below in relation to *gambling.*

In the *Comments* box, you can list any details that help you clarify your answers.

When you think about your worst month* of that behavior in the past year . . .	0 Not at all	1 Some-what	2 A lot	3 A great deal	*Comments?*
1. How much were you "caught up" in the behavior (doing it, thinking about it, etc.)?					
2. How ashamed are/were you about the behavior?					
3. How serious a problem was the behavior?					
4. Did you have losses from the behavior? *(e.g., relationships, job, home, time, money, physical or emotional health, opportunities)*					
5. How successful were you at decreasing the behavior?					
6. How much control did you have over the behavior?					
7. How much did others say you had a problem with the behavior?					
8. Any other sign that the behavior was excessive? List the sign: Rate it on the scale					

*"**Worst month**" means the month in which you were most excessive in the behavior. For example, if your behavior was gambling, it would be the month in the past year in which you spent the most time/money on gambling or had the most severe consequences of gambling (getting into a major fight over it, losing your job over it, etc.). Note that "worst" is not a judgment of you – it is just identifying the most severe month of the behavior, in your opinion.

Step 2: Scoring. The higher your score, the more likely it is that you have a problem with the behavior. This scale is still being researched. For updates, email *info@treatment-innovations.org.*

Step 3: Now go back to your list in Part A, take the next behavior you said Yes or Maybe to, and fill in the same eight-question grid for that behavior. *Continue after that to fill out a grid for each behavior you said Yes or Maybe to in Part A.*

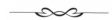

Brief quiz on trauma and addiction

Knowledge is power

This quiz highlights 12 key points on trauma and addiction (but doesn't reflect the contents of the entire book). The answers, with explanations, are at the end.

1. You have to "hit bottom" to recover from addiction. True/False

2. Most people:

   a. Experience trauma

   b. Develop PTSD

   c. Both a and b

   d. Neither a nor b

3. "Many roads, one journey" means there's one path to recovery. True/False

4. You have to tell your trauma story to fully heal. True/False

5. Most people with addiction have an *addictive personality*. True/False

6. Which usually occurs first?

   a. PTSD

   b. Addiction

   c. Both at the same time

   d. Neither

7. No substance or behavior is addictive in and of itself.   True/False

8. Who's more likely to develop PTSD? Those with . . .

    Check all that apply:

    a. Family history of addiction

    b. Severe trauma

    c. Childhood trauma

    d. Repeated trauma

    e. All of the above

9. "Empowerment" means your opinion is right.   True/False

10. To do well in addiction treatment you have to be motivated.   True/False

11. Trauma can increase your risk for all but:

    a. Acute stress disorder

    b. Addiction

    c. Amblyopia

    d. Anxiety

12. To heal from trauma and addiction you must . . .

    Check all that apply:

    a. Decrease your addictive behavior

    b. Forgive others

    c. Tell your trauma story

    d. Attend treatment

    e. All of the above

Quiz answers and explanations

1. You have to "hit bottom" to recover from addiction.   **False**

   Relevance to recovery. Hitting bottom is a wake-up call. It means suffering serious negative consequences from addiction such as losing a job, a partner, or
   your home; getting a DUI; or developing medical problems. Hitting bottom
   is also called *the point of despair*. It does help some people finally accept that
   they have an addiction problem rather than staying in denial. However, many
   people engage in successful recovery without hitting bottom because they
   catch the problem early; this is called *raising the bottom*. See "Find your way"
   (Chapter 9) and "How do people change?" (Chapter 5).

2. Most people:

   a. **Experience trauma**

   b. Develop PTSD

   c. Both a and b

   d. Neither a nor b

   Relevance to recovery. Most people survive one or more traumas in their lifetime. Sadly, trauma is common. Yet most people don't develop PTSD or other
   major problems from it. Feeling upset during or after trauma is common, but
   this usually decreases within 1 to 3 months. Why is this important? It means
   that even if you go through trauma, you may not have lasting problems
   from it. For example, most military personnel who go through trauma typically don't develop PTSD (in part because they're trained to prepare for it in
   advance). Many factors play a role in who develops PTSD. See "It's medical –
   you're not crazy, lazy, or bad" (Chapter 4).

3. "Many roads, one journey" means there's one path   **False**
   to recovery.

   Relevance to recovery. "Many roads, one journey" is a memorable phrase
   conveying that the journey (recovery) can be attained from different paths.
   It's true for both addiction and trauma problems. For example, one person
   might just need self-help groups. Another person might go just to counseling. Another might get medication. Another might do all of these. Choose
   the "roads" that work for you, trying out as many as you can. See "Find your
   way" (Chapter 9).

4. You have to tell your trauma story to fully heal.   **False**

Relevance to recovery. Many people believe this but research shows it's not true. It's a choice, not a requirement. Some people are helped by telling their trauma story, but others find it overly upsetting or unhelpful. Others may want to do it later but aren't ready now; they first want to get their addiction under control, get a job, or get their life on track in some other way first. It's up to you to decide whether and when, if at all, to share your trauma story. You can heal from trauma just as much by staying in the present and focusing on coping skills. See "Two types of trauma counseling" (Chapter 33).

5. Most people with addiction have an *addictive personality*.   **False**

Relevance to recovery. Decades of research indicate that there's no *addictive personality*. Addiction is associated with every personality type: outgoing and reserved; bold and cautious; active and passive. Vulnerability to addiction is based on genetic and social factors and life experiences, but not a specific personality type (see "Find your way," Chapter 9).

6. Which usually occurs first?

   a. PTSD

   b. Addiction

   c. Both at the same time

   d. Neither

Relevance to recovery. Trauma and PTSD usually occur first, then addiction. A major explanation for this pattern is *self-medication* – using addictive behavior for comfort after trauma. It makes sense; people reach out for what helps them feel better, whether it's food, alcohol, gambling, pornography, or any other potentially addictive behavior. That's why this book focuses on finding healthy ways to cope, ways that can sustain you in the long term (see "Why trauma and addiction go together," Chapter 15).

7. No substance or behavior is addictive in and of itself.   **True**

Relevance to recovery. Nothing in and of itself is addictive. Many people use a substance, gamble, shop, work, eat, have sex, and so on without developing a problem. Addiction is caused by a combination of a behavior and a person who's vulnerable to it. Many adolescents and young adults, for example, experiment with substances, but most don't develop an addiction. Most of the adult U.S. population uses alcohol, but only a minority develop alcohol problems. What makes some people more vulnerable to addiction than others? Trauma is one important factor. Other factors include genetics, mental illness, early use of substances, and social influences. Yet some behaviors are more likely to become addictive than others – taking heroin more than eating broccoli, for example (see "Why trauma and addiction go together," Chapter 15).

8. Who's more likely to develop PTSD? Those with . . .

   Check all that apply:

   a. Family history of addiction

   b. Severe trauma

   c. Childhood trauma

   d. Repeated trauma

   e. All of the above

   Relevance to recovery. All trauma isn't equal. For example, rape is more likely to result in PTSD than witnessing a tornado. Traumas that are severe, repeated, forceful, and physically damaging are more likely to result in PTSD than milder traumas. Also, some people are more likely to develop PTSD than others – for example, those with lower education, a lot of stress, mental illness or addiction, and childhood trauma. If you have PTSD, know that you're not alone. There are good reasons you responded the way you did. PTSD has been called "a normal reaction to abnormal events." It's understandable that you may have emotional problems from trauma (see "It's medical – you're not crazy, lazy, or bad," Chapter 4).

9. "Empowerment" means your opinion is right.   **False**

   Relevance to recovery. "Empowerment" means you have the power to choose. But you might still make poor choices. That's why it's important to listen to others, consider your options, and make clear and conscious decisions, not impulsive ones. Most of all, observe your behavior – are you getting better or worse? See "Find your way" (Chapter 9) and "Listen to your behavior" (Chapter 7).

10. To do well in addiction treatment you have to be motivated.   **False**

    Relevance to recovery. It's terrific if you're motivated to reduce addictive behavior – that's the best possible scenario. But motivation may come as a result of recovery efforts rather than at the start of them. Many people find the longer they engage in addiction recovery, the more motivated they are to cut down. Indeed, the National Institute on Drug Abuse has found that people who are forced to attend addiction treatment (mandated) do just as well as those who do so voluntarily (nonmandated). This is encouraging because it means that no matter what your current motivation level is, you can get better (see "Find your way," Chapter 9).

11. Trauma can increase your risk for all but:

   a. Acute stress disorder

   b. Addiction

   c. Amblyopia

   d. Anxiety

Relevance to recovery. Trauma can impact many parts of your life. Acute stress disorder and posttraumatic stress disorder (PTSD) are two mental health problems that can arise from trauma. But trauma also leads to other problems such as addiction, depression, anxiety, physical health problems, social problems (e.g., isolation and distrust), work problems (e.g., poor concentration, legal problems) – but not amblyopia, which is a vision problem known as "lazy eye." Yet remember, too, that you have strengths that trauma does not touch. If you have a sharp sense of humor, artistic abilities, athletic skills – such strengths usually endure. When looking at trauma's impact, honestly notice the problems it creates but also recognize positive qualities that can help your recovery. You're more than your trauma and addiction (see "Starting out," Chapter 2).

12. To heal from trauma and addiction you must . . .

   Check all that apply:

   a. Decrease your addictive behavior

   b. Forgive others

   c. Tell your trauma story

   d. Attend treatment

   e. All of the above

Relevance to recovery. The only required element in the list above is to decrease your addictive behavior. Continuing an addiction makes it harder for you to recover from trauma and creates its own set of addiction-related problems. The earlier you stop or reduce addictive behavior, the better. But nothing else on the list is required for recovery; all are options that some find helpful but not others. For example, you don't have to forgive others (option "b") unless you choose to. Telling your trauma story (option "c") helps some people but not others. Attending counseling (option "d") is encouraged, especially if you have major addiction or trauma problems, but people can recover without professional treatment; they may choose to rely on supportive people, self-help groups, self-help books, and other resources. There are many ways to recover (see "Find your way," Chapter 9, and "Forgiving yourself," Chapter 16).

References

Alcoholics Anonymous. (2004). *Alcoholics Anonymous: The story of how many thousands of men and women have recovered from alcoholism* ["The Big Book"] (4th ed.). New York: Alcoholics Anonymous World Service.

American Psychiatric Association. (2013). *Diagnostic and statistical manual of mental disorders* (5th ed.). Arlington, VA: Author.

Barr, A. (2006). *An investigation into the extent to which psychological wounds inspire counsellors and psychotherapists to become wounded healers, the significance of these wounds on their career choice, the causes of these wounds and the overall significance of demographic factors.* Unpublished master's thesis, University of Strathclyde, Scotland.

Bonds Shapiro, A. (2012). The power of imagery: Can we imagine ourselves well? *Psychology Today.* Retrieved from *www.psychologytoday.com/blog/healing-possibility/201206/the-power-imagery.*

Burroughs, A. (2003). *Dry: A memoir.* New York: St. Martin's Press.

Carnes, P. (2001). *Out of the shadows: Understanding sexual addiction.* Center City, MN: Hazelden.

Cavalcade Productions. (1995). *Counting the cost: The lasting impact of childhood trauma* [Educational video]. Nevada City, CA: Author.

Davis, B. (2006). Psychodynamic psychotherapies and the treatment of co-occurring psychological trauma and addiction. *Journal of Chemical Dependency Treatment, 8*(2), 41–69.

Department of Mental Health and Addiction Services, State of Connecticut. (2000). *Trauma: No more secrets* [Video]. Hartford, CT: Author.

Evans, A. C., Lamb, R., & White, W. L. (2014). *Promoting intergenerational resilience and recovery: Policy, clinical, and recovery support strategies to alter the intergenerational transmission of alcohol, drug, and related problems.* Philadelphia: Philadelphia Department of Behavioral Health and Intellectual Disability Services. Retrieved from *www.williamwhitepapers.com.*

Freire, P. (1970). *Pedagogy of the oppressed.* New York: Continuum.

Foxhall, K. (2001). Learning to live past 9:02 a.m., April 19, 1995. *Monitor on Psychology, 32,* 26.

Goffman, E. (1963). *Stigma: Notes on the management of spoiled identity.* New York: Simon & Schuster.

Goleman, D. (1989, January 24). Sad legacy of abuse: The search for remedies. *The New York Times.* Retrieved from *www.nytimes.com/1989/01/24/science/sad-legacy-of-abuse-the-search-for-remedies.html*; see also the University of Minnesota Longitudinal Study of Risk and Adaptation (*www.cehd.umn.edu/icd/research/parent-child/publications/maltreatment.html*).

Harned, M. S., Korslund, K. E., & Linehan, M. M. (2014). A pilot randomized controlled trial of dialectical behavior therapy with and without the Dialectical Behavior Therapy Prolonged Exposure protocol for suicidal and self-injuring women with borderline personality disorder and PTSD. *Behaviour Research and Therapy, 55,* 7–17.

Harris, M., Fallot, R. D., & Berley, R. W. (2005). Special section on relapse prevention: Qualitative interviews on substance abuse relapse and prevention among female trauma survivors. *Psychiatric Services, 56*(10), 1292–1296.

Herman, J. L. (1992). *Trauma and recovery.* New York: Basic Books.

Hilts, P. (1994, August 2). Is nicotine addictive? It depends on whose criteria you use. *The New York Times.* Retrieved from *www.nytimes.com/1994/08/02/science/is-nicotine-addictive-it-depends-on-whose-criteria-you-use.html*.

James, W. (1958). *Varieties of religious experience: A study in human nature.* New York: Mentor. (Original work published 1902)

Jennings, A., & Ralph, R. O. (1997). *In their own words: Trauma survivors and professionals they trust tell what hurts, what helps, and what is needed for trauma services.* Augusta: Department of Mental Health, Mental Retardation and Substance Abuse Services, State of Maine.

Kasl, C. (1990). *Women, sex, and addictions: A search for love and power.* New York: Harper-Trade.

Khantzian, E. J., & Albanese, M. J. (2008). *Understanding addiction as self-medication: Finding hope behind the pain.* Lanham, MD: Rowman & Littlefield.

Knapp, C. (1997). *Drinking: A love story.* New York: Bantam.

Lamott, A. (1999). *Traveling mercies: Some thoughts on faith.* New York: Anchor Books.

Lamott, A. (2005). *Operating instructions: A journal of my son's first year.* New York: Anchor Books.

Leslie, M. E. (2007). *The breaking the cycle compendium: Vol. 1. The roots of relationship.* Toronto: Mothercraft Press.

Levy, P. (2010). The wounded healer: Part 1. Retrieved from *www.awakeninthedream.com/the-wounded-healer-part-1.*

Luborsky, L., Barber, J. P., Siqueland, L., Johnson, S., Najavits, L. M., Frank, A., et al. (1996). The revised Helping Alliance questionnaire (HAq-II): Psychometric properties. *Journal of Psychotherapy Practice and Research, 5,* 260–271.

Marantz Henig, R. (2004, April 4). The quest to forget. *The New York Times.* Retrieved from *www.nytimes.com/2004/04/04/magazine/the-quest-to-forget.html*.

Markus, H., & Nurius, P. (1986). Possible selves. *American Psychologist, 41*(9), 954.

Marlatt, G., & Gordon, J. (1985). *Relapse prevention: Maintenance strategies in the treatment of addictive behaviors.* New York: Guilford Press.

Miller, D. (2002). Addictions and trauma recovery: An integrated approach. *Psychiatric Quarterly, 73*(2), 157–170. Cited in Morgan, O. J. (2009). Thoughts on the interaction of trauma, addiction, and spirituality. *Journal of Addictions and Offender Counseling, 30*(1), 5–15.

Miller, W. R., Benefield, R. G., & Tonigan, J. S. (1993). Enhancing motivation for change in problem drinking: A controlled comparison of two therapist styles. *Journal of Consulting and Clinical Psychology, 61,* 455–461.

Miller, W. R., & C' de Baca, J. (2001). *Quantum change: When epiphanies and sudden insights transform ordinary lives.* New York: Guilford Press.

Miller, W. R., & White, W. (2007). The use of confrontation in addiction treatment: History, science and time for change. *Counselor: The Magazine for Addiction Professionals, 8*(4), 12–30.

Morgan, O. J. (2009). Thoughts on the interaction of trauma, addiction, and spirituality. *Journal of Addictions and Offender Counseling, 30*(1), 5–15.

Morris, D. J. (2015, January 17). After PTSD, more trauma. *The New York Times.* Retrieved from *http://opinionator.blogs.nytimes.com/2015/01/17/after-ptsd-more-trauma.*

Najavits, L. M. (2002). Clinicians' views on treating posttraumatic stress disorder and substance use disorder. *Journal on Substance Abuse Treatment, 22,* 79–85.

Najavits, L. M. (2002). *Seeking Safety: A treatment manual for PTSD and substance abuse.* New York: Guilford Press.

Najavits, L. M. (2005). *Example of a group session: Asking for help* (Seeking Safety video training series). Newton Centre, MA: Treatment Innovations.

Najavits, L. M. (2010). *Excessive Behavior Scale.* Unpublished manuscript, Treatment Innovations, Newton Centre, MA.

Najavits, L. M. (2014). Creating Change: A new past-focused model for PTSD and substance abuse. In P. Ouimette & J. P. Read (Eds.), *Trauma and substance abuse: causes, consequences, and treatment of comorbid disorders* (pp. 281–303). Washington, DC: American Psychological Association Press.

Najavits, L. M. (forthcoming). *Creating Change: A past-focused treatment manual for trauma, addiction, or both.* New York: Guilford Press.

Najavits, L. M., & Anderson, M. L. (2015). Psychosocial treatments for posttraumatic stress disorder. In P. E. Nathan & J. M. Gorman (Eds.), *A guide to treatments that work* (4th ed., pp. 571–592). New York: Oxford University Press.

Najavits, L. M., & Hien, D. A. (2013). Helping vulnerable populations: A comprehensive review of the treatment outcome literature on substance use disorder and PTSD. *Journal of Clinical Psychology, 69,* 433–480.

Najavits, L. M., Hyman, S. M., Ruglass, L. M., Hien, D. A., & Read, J. P. (2017). Substance use disorder and trauma. In S. Gold, J. Cook, & C. Dalenberg (Eds.), *Handbook of trauma psychology* (pp. 195–214). Washington, DC: American Psychological Association.

National Institute on Drug Abuse. (2012). *Principles of drug addiction treatment: A research-based guide* (3rd ed.). Washington, DC: Author. Retrieved from *www.drugabuse.gov/publications/principles-drug-addiction-treatment-research-based-guide-third-edition/principles-effective-treatment.*

National Institute on Drug Abuse. (2014). *Drugs, brains, and behavior: The science of addiction.* Washington, DC: Author. Retrieved from *www.drugabuse.gov/publications/drugs-brains-behavior-science-addiction/treatment-recovery.*

Neff, K. D. (2003). Development and validation of a scale to measure self-compassion. *Self and Identity, 2,* 223–250.

Ngor, H. (1988). *Haing Ngor: A Cambodian odyssey.* New York: MacMillan.

O'Brien, S. (2004). *The family silver: A memoir of depression and inheritance.* Chicago: University of Chicago Press.

Ouimette, P., & Read, J. P. (Eds.). (2014). *Handbook of trauma, PTSD and substance use disorder comorbidity.* Washington, DC: American Psychological Association Press.

Oyserman, D., Bybee, D., Terry, K., & Hart-Johnson, T. (2004). Possible selves as roadmaps. *Journal of Research in Personality, 38*(2), 130–149.

Palmer, P. J., & Scribner, M. (2007). *The courage to teach guide for reflection and renewal.* San Francisco: Jossey-Bass.

Parent, Jr., D. G. (2012). *The warzone PTSD survivors guide.* North Charleston, SC: Create Space.

Rosenthal, M. (2012). *Before the world intruded: Conquering the past and creating the future, a memoir.* Palm Beach Gardens, FL: Your Life After Trauma.

Rosenthal, M. (2013). Get your brain motivated to recover from PTSD. Retrieved from *www.healthyplace.com/blogs/traumaptsdblog/2013/12/25/how-your-brain-develops-motivation-in-ptsd-recovery.*

Rosenthal, M. (2014). PTSD & anger: Part 1. When we hate happy people. Retrieved from *www.healmyptsd.com/2014/07/ptsd-anger-part-1-when-we-hate-happy-people.html.*

Shaffer, H., LaPlante, D., & Nelson, S. (Eds.). (2012). *American Psychological Association's addiction syndrome handbook.* Washington, DC: American Psychological Association.

Shay, J. (1994). *Achilles in Vietnam: Combat trauma and the undoing of character.* New York: Simon & Schuster.

Siegel, R. K. (1989). *Intoxication: Life in pursuit of artificial paradise.* New York: Dutton.

Stone, R. (2007). *No secrets no lies: How black families can heal from sexual abuse.* New York: Harmony.

Stromberg, G., & Merrill, J. (2007). *The harder they fall: Celebrities tell their real-life stories of addiction and recovery.* Center City, MN: Hazelden.

Tucker, C. (2012). U.S. veterans struggle with pain, stigma of post-traumatic stress: New research aimed at mental health. *The Nation's Health, 42,* 1–12.

van den Blink, H. (2008). Trauma and spirituality. *Reflective Practice: Formation and Supervision in Ministry, 28.*

van der Kolk, B. (2014). *The body keeps the score: Brain, mind, and body in the healing of trauma.* New York: Penguin.

Wayne, J. (2017). Definition of synergy in marketing. Retrieved from *http://smallbusiness.chron.com/definition-synergy-marketing-21786.html.*

Weiss, R., & Schneider, J. R. (2015). *Always turned on: Sex addiction in the digital age.* Carefree, AZ: Gentle Path Press.

White, W. L. (2014). Recovery conversion. Retrieved from *www.williamwhitepapers.com/blog/2014/11/recovery-conversion.html.*

Wilson, P. (2013). Two kinds of hope. Retrieved from *www.petewilson.tv/2013/09/25/two-kinds-of-hope.*

Index

Abstinence, 9, 65, 67, 108, 120, 143–144. *See also* Addiction; Treatment
violation effect, 147
Accelerated resolution therapy. *See* Trauma, counseling, past-focused
Addiction, 3–4, 28–33, 103–104. *See also* Behavioral addictions; Relapse, addiction; Trauma and addiction
craving, 127
resources, 252–253
severity (mild, moderate, severe), 3, 17, 30, 33, 68, 109, 144
signs of, 32–33
exercise, 33
substances, 4, 30–31, 103, 104–105, 108, 122, 150
urine testing, 42, 68
vulnerability, 103–106, 118, 122
Anger, 125, 130, 159, 187–191, 208, 226. *See also* Feelings, negative

B

Behavioral addictions, 4, 29, 31, 33, 158. *See also* Addiction
Beyond trauma. *See* Trauma, counseling, present-focused
Binge eating disorder. *See* Behavioral addictions

Biology. *See* Trauma and addiction, physical aspects
Body. *See also* Trauma and addiction, physical aspects
exercise, 122–123
Brain changes, 31, 92, 117, 118, 120, 181
Brief eclectic psychotherapy. *See* Trauma, counseling
Brief quiz on trauma and addiction, 261–267

C

Calming. *See* Grounding
Change, methods of, 35–44
Coercion, 41
Cognitive-behavioral therapy, 68. *See also* Trauma, counseling
Cognitive processing therapy. *See* Trauma, counseling, past-focused
Compassion, 15, 34, 36, 64, 68, 97–101. *See also* Forgiveness
exercise, 101
toward oneself, 99–100
toward others, 100
Concurrent treatment of PTSD and SUD using prolonged exposure. *See* Trauma, counseling
Controlled use, 9, 65, 68, 144. *See also* Addiction; Treatment

Conversion, 37–39
Coping, 35–36. *See also* Safe coping
Creativity, 43. *See also* Imagery; Imagination
Culture of silence. *See* Silencing

D

Depressants. *See* Addiction, substances
Dialectical behavior therapy, 215, 218.
  See Trauma, counseling, present-focused
Dissociation, 26, 125, 242–243

E

Electronic addictions. *See* Behavioral
  addictions
Emotion. *See* Feelings, negative
Emotional freedom techniques. *See* Trauma,
  counseling, past-focused
Empowerment, 61–62
Excessive Behavior Scale, 256–260
Exercise addiction. *See* Behavioral addictions
Exposure therapy. *See* Trauma, counseling,
  past-focused
Eye movement desensitization and
  reprocessing therapy. *See* Trauma,
  counseling, past-focused

F

Family history, 27, 107, 110, 122, 150–154
Feelings, negative, 186–193
  strategies for, 188–193
Forgiveness, 112–115. *See also* Compassion
  exercise, 114–115

G

Gambling addiction, 103, 106, 117, 141.
  See Behavioral addictions
Goffman, Erving, 173
Grief, 37–38, 189

Grounding, 125–130
 definition, 125
 exercise, 129–130
 guidelines, 126, 128–129
 methods, 127–129

H

Hallucinogens. *See* Addiction, substances
Harm reduction, 9, 68, 143–144, 252. *See*
  also Addiction; Treatment
Harm (to self or others), 4, 12–13, 117, 126,
  158, 193
Helpers, advice for, 231–249. *See*
  also Wounded healer
 dilemmas, 232, 239–240
 dos and don'ts, 236–238
 education, 235–236
 emergency plan, 243–244. *See also* Suicide
  prevention
 rewards of helping, 246
 strategies, 235–246
Helping Alliance Questionnaire, Revised,
  209–210
Helping others, 43, 177, 190–191. *See*
  also Wounded healer
HIV/AIDS, resources, 254–255

I

Identity, 72–76, 166–170
 exercise, 74–76
Imagery, 196–197, 198, 201–204. *See*
  also Imagination
 exercise, 203–204
Imagery rehearsal therapy. *See* Trauma,
  counseling, present-focused
Imagination, 195–199. *See also* Imagery
 exercise, 195–199
Integrated cognitive-behavioral therapy
  for PTSD and alcohol use disorder.
  See Trauma, counseling

L

Language, 11–12, 78–85
  addiction, 79–81
  exercise, 79–83
  trauma, 81–83
Learning, new, 45–46, 179–185
  exercise, 181–183, 227–229

M

Medical. *See also* Physical
  information, searching, 255
  problems/conditions, 17, 24–35, 117,
    119–120, 189, 256
Moderation Management, 68
Motivation, 64, 65, 136–139
  exercise, 138–139

O

Opioids. *See* Addiction, substances

P

Physical
  change, 40
  problems. *See* Medical, problems
Pink cloud, 47
Possible selves. *See* Identity
Present-centered therapy. *See* Trauma,
  counseling, present-focused

R

Rage. *See* Anger
Rational recovery, 243
Recovery, 72. *See also* Imagery; Imagination;
    Resources
  exercise, 142–146, 227–229
  goals, 143–144
  identity, 168–171

inspiration, 45–46
plan for increasing, 141–148
signs of being in, 6, 72–73, 226–227
signs of not being in, 6, 73–74
Relapse, 121, 147, 155–157. *See also* Pink cloud
  addiction, 155–156
  prevention, 68
  trauma problems, 156
Resilience-oriented treatment for PTSD.
    See Trauma, counseling
Resources, 45–46, 250–255
Rethinking Drinking, 30, 64, 68, 253

S

Safe Behavior Scale, 51–54
Safe coping, 33–35, 48–50, 86–89. *See
    also* Coping
  exercise, 48–49
  rehearsal, 162–165
    exercise, 162–163
  Safe Coping Skills List, 86–89
Safety, 48, 196, 198. *See also* Safe coping;
    Suicide prevention
  behavior, 48–51, 142–146. *See also* Excessive
      Behavior Scale; Safe Behavior Scale
Seeking Safety therapy, 68, 86, 215. *See
    also* Trauma, counseling, present-focused
Self-compassion. *See* Compassion
Self-forgiveness. *See* Forgiveness
Self-fulfilling prophecy, 175
Sex/pornography addiction. *See* Behavioral
    addictions
Sexual problems, 119
Shopping/spending addiction. *See* Behavioral
    addictions
Silencing, 131–135
Skills training in affect and interpersonal
    regulation/exposure therapy.
    See Trauma, counseling
Slip. *See* Relapse
SMART Recovery, 10, 65, 223, 243, 253
Social messages, 150–154, 181
  exercise, 151–153
Social mission. *See* Helping others

Social pain, 91–95. *See also* Stigma
Spirituality, 61, 68, 126, 223
Splitting, 168
Stigma, 95, 172–178. *See also* Social pain
    strategies for overcoming, 175–177
Stimulants. *See* Addiction, substances
Stress, 3, 107, 121, 125, 156, 159, 160, 190, 201
Stress inoculation training. *See* Trauma,
    counseling, present-focused
Suicide prevention, resources, 253–254

T

Testimony therapy, 223. *See* Trauma,
    counseling, past-focused
Trauma, 2–3, 25–28. *See also* Trauma and
    addiction
    counseling, 214–221
        exercise, 214–215, 218–220
        past-focused, 67, 216–217
        present-focused, 67, 215–216
    definition, 2
    problems/symptoms, 25–29. *See
        also* Relapse, trauma problems
        exercise, 28
    resources, 250–252
Trauma affect regulation: guide for education
    and therapy. *See* Trauma, counseling,
    present-focused
Trauma and addiction, 4–10, 15, 104–111. *See
    also* Brief quiz on trauma and addiction
    exercise, 109–111, 158–161
    identity, 167–168
    linkages, 158–161
        exercise, 158–161
    perception by others, 172–173
    physical aspects, 117–123
    social messages, 150–154, 180–181
    treatment, 68–69
Trauma-informed care, 67

Trauma management therapy. *See* Trauma,
    counseling
Trauma recovery and empowerment model
    therapy. *See* Trauma, counseling, present-
    focused
Traumatic brain injury, 120, 190
Treatment, 63–71. *See also* Trauma,
    counseling; Trauma and addiction,
    treatment
    counselor, selection of, 206–2132. *See
        also* Helping Alliance Questionnaire,
        Revised
    evidence-based, 69
    exercise, 69–71
    types (integrated, parallel, sequential), 68
Triggers, 16, 121, 127, 147–148, 187, 215, 224,
    242
Truth, facing, 55–59
    exercise, 59
12-step groups, 33, 65, 66, 223, 235, 243,
    252–253

U

Urine testing, 42

V

Virtual reality therapy. *See* Trauma,
    counseling, past-focused

W

Women for Sobriety, 243
Work addiction. *See* Behavioral addictions
Wounded healer, 222–225. *See also* Helping
    others

About the Author

Lisa M. Najavits, PhD, is Adjunct Professor of Psychiatry at the University of Massachusetts Medical School and Director of Treatment Innovations, LLC, which conducts research and training related to mental health and addiction. She served on the faculty of Harvard Medical School for 25 years and Boston University School of Medicine and Veterans Affairs Boston Healthcare System for 12 years. An award-winning clinician and researcher, Dr. Najavits is author of *Seeking Safety: A Treatment Manual for PTSD and Substance Abuse*, a bestselling book for mental health professionals.